Handbook of Clinical Psychopharmacology for Therapists

John Preston, Psy.D.
John H. O'Neal, M.D.
Mary C. Talaga, B.S., Pharm., R.Ph., M.A.

New Harbinger Publications, Inc.

Publisher's Note

This publication is designed to provide accurate and authoritative information in regard to the subject matter covered. It is sold with the understanding that the publisher is not engaged in rendering psychological, financial, legal, or other professional services. If expert assistance or counseling is needed, the services of a competent professional should be sought.

To the best of our knowledge, recommended doses of medications listed in this book are accurate. However, they are not meant to serve as a guide for prescribing of medications. Physicians, please check the manufacturer's product information sheet or the *Physicians' Desk Reference* for any changes in dosage schedule or contraindications.

Figures 5-A, 5-B, 5-E, 7-D, 7-E, 8-B, and 14-F have been previously published in *Clinical Psychopharmacology Made Ridiculously Simple*, 1994, MedMaster Inc., Miami, and are reproduced here with the permission of the copyright holder.

*To my boys, Matt and David—*J. P.

*To Wendy, Sean, and Matthew for their loving support through the writing of this book—*J. O.

*To my parents for opening my mind . . . and to my sons for opening my heart—*M. T.

What is paraded as scientific fact is simply the current belief of some scientists. We are accustomed to regard science as truth with a capital "T". What scientific knowledge is, in fact, is the best available approximation of truth in the judgment of the majority of scientists who work in the particular specialty involved. Truth is not something that we possess, it is a goal towards which we hopefully strive ... the current opinion of the scientific establishment is only the latest and never the last word.

—M. Scott Peck, M.D.,
author of *The Road Less Traveled*

Contents

Acknowledgments

Many thanks to our publisher, Dr. Matthew McKay, and our editor, Leslie Tilley, for helping our ideas to take form. To Laurie Barrall and the Wet Ink Crew, as usual, a job well done! Appreciation also goes to Diana Jackson and the folks at Exact Copy.

To our families and friends, with deep appreciation, for their patience and encouragement throughout this project.

Finally, heartfelt thanks to our students and our patients. May this book reach many and hopefully contribute to our ongoing struggle to reduce emotional suffering.

Part One

Understanding Psychopharmacology: The Basics

Part one of this book briefly covers the development of psychopharmacology from a historical and sociological perspective and then goes on to provide an overview of neurochemistry and biological-psychological functioning. The purpose of these chapters is not to provide a comprehensive discussion of the fields of pharmacology or physiology, but is simply to familiarize you with the basic terminology and models of pharmacokinetics.

1

Introduction

This book is intended primarily for mental health professionals and those in graduate training in psychology, social work, and counseling. The professional goal of most readers will be to provide services that aim to reduce emotional pain, to promote psychological growth and healing, and to foster the development of personal autonomy. To this end, we in the field are trained in various theoretical approaches that attempt to explain the development of maladaptive lifestyles and subjectively painful psychiatric symptoms. These theories serve to give meaning and coherence to what we do in clinical practice and, most importantly, lay a foundation of understanding so that interventions make sense and further the goal of reducing suffering in ways that are effective.

Many schools of thought exist regarding the origins of mental health problems. As has been well documented in the history of psychiatry, as schools of thought evolve, controversy, dogma, and empassioned belief systems emerge. It may be inherent to the development and maturation of science that these emotionally toned belief systems and the resulting debates occur.

Most recently, from the mid-sixties through the seventies, polarization occurred within psychiatry between those advocating psychological theories (primarily psychodynamic and behavioral models) and those on the other side of the fence (using biological and medical models). The disagreements that emerged were more than differences of opinion or dry debate. Each school attracted followers who had strong emotional investments in their perspective.

For many years this division resulted in the development of barriers between groups of mental health clinicians—and at times in fragmentation in care. Fortunately, during the past decade something has changed. We are beginning to witness a shift in thinking, as increasing numbers of practitioners and training institutes move away from egocentric and dogmatic positions and begin to embrace a more integrated approach with regard to both theories of etiology and methods of treatment.

New discoveries in the neurosciences, refined technical advances in psychotherapy, and a large number of outcome studies in both pharmacotherapy and psychotherapy have made it abundantly clear: People are complex. Mental health problems spring from many sources; and reductionist, unidimentional models are simply inadequate to explain the wide array of mental and emotional problems people experience. Likewise, no single approach to treatment works for all problems. Certain disorders clearly respond better to certain interventions, whereas others require alternative approaches.

In writing this book, although our primary focus is on psychopharmacology, we share a strong respect for what will be termed *integrative approaches* to treatment: recognition of the importance of varied treatments and collaboration among professionals from different disciplines.

We hope that you will find this book helpful as you engage in this most important profession and work toward the goal of reducing emotional pain.

History of Biological Psychiatry

In understanding psychopharmacology, it may be helpful if you are able to place it in a historical context. Let's take a brief look at this history as it unfolded.

In the late 1800s psychiatry was clearly rooted in the medical model and the neurology of the day. Psychiatrists believed, almost exclusively, that mental illness could be attributed to some sort of biologic disturbance. The earliest attempts to approach the understanding of mental illness in this era, involved two main areas of investigation.

On one front was the development of the first systematic nosologic system by Emil Kraepelin. This pioneering work laid the foundation for all later diagnostic schema (such as the *Diagnostic and Statistical Manual of Mental Disorders*, or *DSM*). And many of Kraepelin's original notions about the classification of major mental illness have stood the test of time. He was a brilliant investigator and the one most responsible for ushering in descriptive clinical psychiatry. However, his endeavors must have been accompanied by a good deal of frustration and impotence, since, despite the development of a systematic approach to diagnosis, Kraepelin and other psychiatrists of his time had few if any methods of treatment.

At the same time, the hunt was on for evidence of brain pathology, which was presumed to underlie mental illness. Research was conducted in neuroanatomy labs but yielded few concrete results. For example, the famous French neurologist Jean-Martin Charcot believed that hysterical conversation symptoms were undoubtedly due to some type of central nervous system lesion. He explained the fact that no demonstrable pathology could be isolated on autopsy by saying it simply suggested that somehow the lesion mysteriously disappeared at the time of death. We must bear in mind, however, that in all likelihood, these researchers and clinicians were desperate to find causes and cures and went at it by the means best known to them (biology) and using the scant technology available at the time.

Biological psychiatry got a shot in the arm in the late 1800s, as two discoveries were made. At the time, probably one half of those housed in asylums suffered from a type of psychotic-organic brain syndrome which ultimately was found to be caused by the *Treponema pallidum* bacteria (a central nervous system infection seen in the late stages of syphilis). It was also eventually discovered that some organic mental syndromes were due to pellagra (a disease associated with niacin and protein deficiency). These were important discoveries, and they fueled enthusiasm in biological psychiatrists. It was just a matter of time, they felt, before other biologic causes would be isolated and medical treatments developed. However, such discoveries did not occur until the middle of the twentieth century. For practical purposes, biological psychiatry came to a halt as it entered the 1900s.

The disappointments stemming from medical research on mental illness and the failure to develop any effective treatment probably increased the receptivity of psychiatry to divergent approaches. At this same time Sigmund Freud was assembling the basic notions of psychoanalysis. Freud's initial theory was strongly influenced by his own medical and neurological training (for example, his "Project for a Scientific Psychology," 1895), and many of his prevailing ideas continued to have their roots in biology, including drive theory, instincts, and psychosexual development. However, his newly emerging theory and techniques of treatment sparked interest in the use of novel, nonmedical approaches to treatment.

By the 1920s psychological (rather than biological) explanations for the development and treatment of psychopathology had found their place in clinical psychiatry, and by the 1940s psychodynamic thinking had permeated American psychiatry and become the dominant theoretical model. Yet these newly developed approaches proved to be inadequate in the treatment of the more serious forms of mental illness, such as schizophrenia and manic-depressive psychosis. In one of his last manuscripts, Freud himself admitted his disappointment in psychoanalytic methods for treating schizophrenia. He hypothesized that eventually it would be discovered that these grave mental disorders were due to some form of biologic abnormality, and that perhaps drugs would eventually be found to treat these illnesses.

Somatic Therapies

In the days of Kraepelin, pharmaceuticals were used to treat mentally ill patients. Generally, the drugs were prescribed to sedate wildly agitated psychotic patients. For example, Kraepelin listed in one of his textbooks the following group of recommended medications (Spiegel and Aebi 1989):

For Agitation	To Produce Sleep
Opium	Chloral Hydrate
Morphine	Ether
Scopolamine	Alcohol
Hashish	Chloroform
	Bromides

Kraepelin noted, however, that none of these preparations cured mental illness, that they were for short-term use, and that a number of them could lead to problems with addiction. All of these drugs achieved behavioral control by sedating patients; none really affected psychotic symptoms per se, nor did they have any impact on activating patients who were stuporous or clinically depressed.

Other somatic therapies were developed in the first half of the twentieth century, with variable results. Malaria therapy was conceived in 1917, insulin shock in 1927, psychosurgery in 1936, and electroconvulsive treatment (ECT) in 1938. All of these methods, as originally conceived, carried serious risks, and most demonstrated marginal effectiveness. Psychosurgeries were carried out by the thousands in the 1940s, resulting in rather effective behavioral control over agitated psychotic patients but at great human cost. Many, if not most lobotomized patients were reduced to anergic, passive, and emotionally dead human beings.

Electroconvulsive treatment conversely, was quite effective in certain groups of patients, such as those with psychotic depressive disorders. However, early methods of administration were fraught with dangerous complications and side effects, and ECT was used on a widespread basis, indiscriminately. Many patients were treated with it inappropriately and did not respond. (As shall be discussed later, in recent years significant advances have been made in ECT, and it now affords a highly effective, safe treatment for selected types of patients.)

Most severely ill patients in the late nineteenth and early twentieth centuries continued to be housed in overcrowded state mental hospitals and were "treated" using tried and true methods of the day: seclusion, restraint, and wet sheet packs. Although seemingly inhumane procedures were employed, it may be important to consider that the psychiatrists of that era were relatively helpless in the face of very severe mental illnesses and that these approaches (although certainly misused at times) reflected their attempt to reduce the horrendous human suffering seen in thousands of severely ill people.

New Discoveries

In the 1950s, three new discoveries heralded the beginnings of a new interest in biological psychiatry. Interestingly, these three areas of investigation were conducted by separate groups of researchers, each with little knowledge of the work being done by their colleagues. (Kety 1975).

Thorazine and other early psychotropic drugs

Immediately after World War II, medical researchers and chemists working for pharmaceutical companies were trying to develop a drug that would reduce the complications associated with shock following major surgery. In early 1951, a compound initially labeled #4560 RP was developed and testing with surgical patients was begun (Spiegel and Aebi 1989). The initial results were encouraging. Given preoperatively, it was able to relax patients, somewhat reduced postoperative shock, and proved to be a good antiemetic (preventing postsurgical nausea). The finding that it produced noticeable sedation came as a surprise. In the aftermath of field trials with surgical patients, the pharmaceutical company Laborit decided to try this medication with restless, agitated psychiatric patients to help improve sleep, totally unaware that the drug would prove to have more widespread effects on the psychiatric patients that were tested.

Initial clinical trials first reported in 1952, resulted in marked behavioral changes when given to manic and schizophrenic patients. Not only did it produce a calming effect, but after a period of time it actually appeared to reduce psychotic symptoms such as delusions and hallucinations. Additional studies were carried out the following year, and by 1954 the drug was approved for use. The new medication was given the generic name chlorpromazine; in the United States it was marketed under the brand name Thorazine. It received immediate acceptance, and by the end of 1954, for the first time ever, there was a marked decrease in the number of patients incarcerated in state mental hospitals: the first major breakthrough in psychopharmacology.

Other psychotropic medications were discovered during the fifties. The first antidepressant was developed in 1952 (iproniazid, an MAO inhibitor), although clinical studies in humans did not take place until 1956. The first tricyclic antidepressant, imipramine (Tofranil), was developed in 1954 and entered the market in 1957. The first minor tranquilizer, meprobamate, was released in 1955, followed shortly by the safer benzodiazepine, chlordiazepoxide (Librium) in 1958. Finally, lithium carbonate, originally used as a sedative by J. Cade in 1948, began to be used to treat manic-depressive illness in the early 1960s.

It is interesting to note that most of these psychopharmacological discoveries were accidental; that is, the drug companies were developing medications to treat other, medical illnesses, and just happened to find that the drugs could affect psychiatric symptoms. Also, these discoveries were made empirically; they were not developed as an outgrowth of a particular theory of neurochemical dysfunction, nor was the mechanism of action at all known. What was evident was that the medications worked and were far superior to any previous treatments for severe mental illness.

The synapse and neurochemical transmission

Although C. S. Sherrington inferred the existence of the synapse (the small space separating individual nerve cells) as early as 1906, the specific details of synaptic transmission were not fully understood for many decades thereafter. Sherrington's ideas involved a sort of telephone switchboard model of the nervous system, and neuronal messages were assumed to be transmitted via electrical stimulation. It was not until the 1950s that neuroscientists realized that communication between nerve cells, although partially electrochemical in nature, is largely due to the release of chemical substances. These chemicals, which transmit energy from one nerve cell to another, are referred to as neurotransmitters; other chemicals that play an indirect role in neurotransmission are called neuromodulators.

With this discovery, it became possible to imagine that certain neurologic dysfunctions might be caused by chemical irregularities and, that therefore it might be possible to develop drugs that could influence or alter neurotransmitter function.

Genetic studies

The third line of investigation involved both genetics and studies of familial patterns of mental illness. The earliest research in this direction was ultimately criticized for numerous methodological flaws. Yet some of the basic findings proved to be fundamentally correct. There is a strong genetic loading for certain mental illnesses, in particular for schizophrenia and manic-depressive illness. (In recent times evidence has been obtained revealing genetic loadings for a number of mental disorders, although clearly the strongest evidence exists for bipolar disorder and some types of schizophrenia.)

Controversy

By the early sixties then, it had been discovered that synaptic activation is chemical in nature; certain illnesses seem to be genetically passed on from generation to generation (and genetic factors are expressed biochemically); and newer drugs could significantly reduce psychiatric symptoms. The triangulation of this data provided rather strong support for a renewed interest in biological psychiatry. There was new hope for the millions of patients suffering from serious mental illness, and psychiatry had begun to step back into "real medicine" again.

However, despite the advances, these new treatments were plagued by a host of side effects—some unpleasant, some actually dangerous. These potent drugs were also often overused or were misused in certain treatment settings. Consequently, controversy began to arise, both among professionals, and in the lay public and mass media.

Professional dissention

Within professional ranks, debate issued from two fairly discrete theoretical camps: those who were pro-medication and those who were pro-psychotherapy. Each group amassed impassioned arguments not only in favor of their own point of view, but also against the other school of thought, as set out below.

Pro-medication (anti-psychotherapy)—arguments in favor of medication treatment, as the treatment of choice:

- Because of its quantifiable nature—that is, the ability to monitor dosage—medication treatment can be studied much more systematically than psychotherapy.

- Medications act quickly to reduce painful and debilitating symptoms.

- The quicker response seen with medications can help to restore hope and reduce demoralization.

- Treatment with medications can be conducted in a much more systematic and standardized fashion, whereas psychotherapy relies heavily on the individual skill of the psychotherapist.

- Rapid and effective symptom relief can potentially reduce suffering to such an extent that the patient is better able to engage productively in psychotherapy. Likewise, the reductions of drive strength afforded by some psychotropic medications may operate to free up more psychic energy, which could then be channeled into adaptive ego functions.

- Medications can provide help to patients who have limited intellectual capacity, poor ego strength, or both; that is, drugs may be effective with people for whom psychotherapy is inappropriate.

- Psychotherapy is often prolonged and expensive, may be unavailable to many people, and is of unproven effectiveness (this was the case especially in light of the very limited psychotherapy outcome studies available in the 1950s and 1960s). Thus medications are much more cost-effective and more readily available to the general public.

Finally, those strongly wedded to a biochemical model of psychopathology contended that social, behavioral, and psychological approaches simply could not correct the underlying biologic abnormality responsible for major mental illnesses. Recent studies, however, have cast doubt on this hypothesis.

Pro-psychotherapy (anti-medication)—arguments in favor of psychotherapy as the treatment of choice:

- Only psychotherapy, not medications, can address the complexity of human psychological functioning. Medications only treat symptoms, whereas psychotherapy focuses on the whole person or psyche.

- Psychotherapy aims toward personal growth and autonomy, whereas drugs are likely to foster dependency, either on the doctor or on the drug itself.

- Drugs can interfere with autonomy and expressions of free will, whereas psychotherapy honors these processes. The prescription of medications may, at least at an unconscious level, communicate the message that the drug will do the work, you don't have to. (Numerous documented instances of overuse of tranquilizing medications to achieve behavioral control provided fodder for this argument.)

- Medications may reduce anxiety and other forms of suffering to such an extent that people will be less motivated to engage in psychotherapy.

- Many drugs have undesirable or dangerous side effects, and some can lead to dependence and abuse.

- Medications ultimately do not solve problems, teach adaptive coping skills, mend broken hearts, or fill empty lives (Menninger 1963).

Although this debate continued throughout the 1960s and 1970s, clearly there were also a number of what G. L. Klerman (Beitman and Klerman 1991) calls "pragmatic practitioners"—those mental health professionals that used whatever approaches seemed to work. Certainly it was, and is, reasonable to consider that some disorders are best treated by psychotropic medications, others by psychotherapy, and it often makes sense to use a combination of both modalities.

Public opinion

A parallel to the professional debate began to occur within the general public. In institutes of higher education, the humanistic movement began to permeate not only departments of psychology but the global academic community as well. The post-McCarthy social climate was ripe for new attitudes that challenged political and social control and applauded the expression of free will, self-expression, and self-actualization. Reports began to surface regarding the abuse of psychiatric medication by the medical profession. Opponents to drug treatment accused the psychiatrists of using medications to achieve control. The term "chemical straightjacket" became popularized.

The 1970s saw the proliferation of new tranquilizers, and pharmaceutical companies reaped fortunes from the sale of well-known pills such as Valium and Librium. The vast majority of prescriptions written for minor tranquilizers (more than 90 percent) were written by family practice doctors, not psychiatric specialists. The "drugged state" was the fastest growing state in the union (Bly 1990). The inappropriate use and abuse of tranquilizers gained increasing public attention and even found its way into popular songs (the Rolling Stones' "Mother's Little Helper") and movies (*I'm Dancing As Fast As I Can*).

In the 1960s, the Church of Scientology was successfully sued by the American Psychiatric Association. In retaliation, it began a long, embittered assault on American psychiatry. Initially the Church of Scientology launched a negative campaign against the use of Ritalin, a psychotropic medication used to treat attention-deficit disorder. More recently it has orchestrated a move to shed negative light on the antidepressant Prozac (see sidebar).

Biological psychiatry was under attack. Although clearly there was a good deal of abuse and misuse of psychoactive drugs, there also continued to be decreasing numbers of people living in mental hospitals, and drug companies were at work developing newer and "cleaner" psychotropic medications, medications with fewer side effects.

Medications and the Media

Research studies and clinical experience certainly influence prescribing practices. However, in recent years the media has had a profound effect on public opinion and ultimately on clinical practice.

In the late 1980s negative attention was focused on the drug Ritalin (methylphenidate), a widely prescribed stimulant used in the treatment of hyperactivity and attention deficit disorder (ADD). Andrew Brotman, summarizing the work of Safer and Krager (1992) states "The media attack was lead by major national television talk show hosts and in the opinion of the authors, allowed anecdotal and unsubstantiated allegations concerning Ritalin to be aired. There were also over twenty lawsuits initiated throughout the country, most by a lawyer linked to the Church of Scientology." (Brotman 1992).

In a study of the effects of this negative media and litigation blitz conducted in Baltimore County, Maryland, Safer and Krager (1992) found that the use of Ritalin had dropped significantly. From 1981 through 1987, the use of Ritalin had increased fivefold. However, in the two-year period during and just following the negative media attention, there was a 40 percent decrease in prescriptions for Ritalin. And this decrease occurred at a time when research on ADD and stimulant treatment continued to strongly support the safety and efficacy of such medications. The authors go on to state that 36 percent of children who discontinued Ritalin experienced major academic maladjustment (such as failing grades or being suspended), and an additional 47 percent who discontinued encountered

continued

Rapprochement: Biological and Psychological Perspectives

During the 1980s, a shift began in which increasing numbers of mental health practitioners and researchers widened their previously narrow views on etiology and treatment of mental illness. Increasingly, it became recognized that unidimensional models, whether psychological or biological, fell short of explaining the tremendous complexities of human psychological functioning and psychopathology. This transition to more complimentary and integrated views of cause and cure can be attributed to several new developments:

- The side effects of medications historically resulted in very poor compliance rates among psychiatric patients, and the most effective medication available is useless if the patient doesn't take the drug as prescribed. Newly discovered compounds introduced in the 1980s and early nineties have yielded effective medications with much more "user-friendly" side effect profiles.

- Discoveries have been made in which new medications and newer uses for existing medications provide very good results in treating certain types of mental illnesses, such as panic disorder and obsessive-compulsive disorder. This greatly increases the psychiatrist's arsenal of effective medications.

- A growing body of well-controlled research studies (double-blind, randomized, placebo controlled) lend convincing support to the efficacy of psychotropic drugs.

- Newly developed neuro-imaging techniques, such as PET and SPECT scans, allow researchers to view metabolic activity in the living brain. These technologies have been able to isolate localized brain abnormalities in certain mental disorders, including panic disorder, schizophrenia, ADD, and obsessive-compulsive disorder. They can provide data on particular sites of drug action or binding and can illustrate changes between the pre- and post-treatment status of particular brain structures. Imaging techniques have added considerable "hard data" to various theories of biochemical etiology in selected mental illnesses.

- Neuro-imaging techniques have been accompanied by a host of new laboratory procedures that allow neuroscientists to assay the neurochemical by-products found in blood, urine, and spinal fluid. Although early psychopharmacology was implemented without any real knowledge of the underlying pathophysiology, in the past decade biochemical theories have gained tremendous scientific support.

These new developments in psychiatry and the neurosciences have been hard to ignore. Many formerly hard-line psychotherapists have been won over by the flood of research findings and their personal experiences in treating people with psychoactive drugs.

During this same period, important advances were made in the theory and practice of psychotherapy. During the late seventies and the eighties the first truly well-controlled psychotherapy studies emerged (including the now popular meta-analyses). The results of these studies cast doubt on the findings of early research that had suggested that psychotherapy was ineffective (Eysenck 1965, for example). Of the many forms of psychotherapy that have been developed, the meta-analyses suggest that no single school of therapy is clearly superior and that psychotherapies across the board are often much more effective than no treatment.

Also during this time we witnessed the development of novel treatment approaches, such as cognitive-behavioral psychotherapy (Beck 1976) and interpersonal psychotherapy (Klerman, et al. 1984) as a treatment for particular disorders, such as depression and panic disorder. These approaches have appeal, in that they can be somewhat systematically applied (some even provide "canned" formats or "cookbooks"). Also, the methodology is a *bit* less reliant on the personal characteristics of the therapist. These approaches then lend themselves to a short-term format and can often be conducted in groups. And, finally, these psychotherapies can be more easily studied. Both cognitive-behavioral and interpersonal psychotherapies have a solid track record of effectiveness (as is discussed further in the next chapter).

Finally, both clinical-anecdotal and research studies have emerged that support the combined use of pharmacotherapy and psychotherapy in the treatment of paricular disorders. At times, the combined treatments have been shown to be superior to either single treatment alone.

mild to moderate academic problems. Concurrently, as Ritalin use (especially new prescriptions) decreased, there was a significant (fourfold) increase in the prescription of tricyclic antidepressants among ADD children. It is important to note that tricyclics, although often used to treat ADD, tend to have more troublesome side effects than Ritalin, and have been implicated in four reports of cardiac fatalities. Brotman (1992) concludes "When there are reports in the media that lead to stigmatization of a certain drug . . . there tends to be a move to other medications which have less notoriety, even if they may, in fact, be more problematic."

More recently, following wide acclaim as a new "breakthrough drug for depression" (Cowley et al. 1990), Prozac (fluoxetine) came under attack by consumer groups and, again, the Church of Scientology. The negative attention was sparked by a single article (Teicher, Glod, and Cole 1990) documenting the emergence or reemergence of suicidal ideas in six patients treated with Prozac. The six patients had been diagnosed as suffering from severe depressive disorders, and in no case were there actual suicide attempts following the onset of treatment with Prozac. But suddenly Prozac was thrust into a very unfavorable light and was the next drug in line to find itself the topic of television talk shows.

Subsequent studies have failed to find any evidence that Prozac is more likely to be associated with suicidal feelings than any other antidepressant (Fava and Rosenbaum 1991; Beasley and Dornseif 1991). In fact, in one study the incidence of suicidal ideations was greater in patients treated

continued

by placebo or imipramine (a tricyclic antidepressant) than by Prozac (Beasley and Dornseif 1991).

The Church of Scientology attempted to convince the Federal Drug Administration (FDA) to pull Prozac from the market. However, the FDA ruled against taking such action because there was no scientific evidence to support the claims made by the Church of Scientology (Burton 1991).

All medications produce some side effects. Reports of adverse effects, even if very infrequent, must be taken seriously and investigated systematically. There is a place for skepticism and scrutiny. However, one must consider the negative effect of unsubstantiated reports in the lay press. For example, the risk of Prozac-induced suicide appears to be *extremely* low, and, the suicide rate in untreated major depression is reported to be 15 percent. Clearly, failure to treat carries the graver risk.

It is very likely that many seriously depressed people and parents of ADD children have been understandably, and unnecessarily, frightened by negative, sensationalistic reports in the media. To quote Brotman (1992) again, "Pharmacotherapy does not exist in a social and political vacuum."

For many in the mental health community, the writing on the wall has become far more legible: A single model for understanding and treating mental disorders is too narrow and is simply inadequate. As we shall be discussing in subsequent chapters, current evidence suggests that particular disorders do respond best to certain medical treatments, and for these, medications are the treatment of choice. Other disorders have little to do with biochemical dysfunction, and medications play little or no role in their treatment. And still other disorders require the skillful integration of biological and psychotherapies.

As the saying goes, when you only have a hammer, every problem looks like a nail. Fortunately, at the present time mental health professionals have access to a "toolbox" of approaches that can, if employed appropriately, dramatically increase our effectiveness in reducing emotional suffering and promoting mental health.

Why Learn About Psychopharmacology?

In the United States, the majority of mental health services are provided by nonmedical therapists. Likewise, the majority of prescriptions for psychotropic medications are written by family practice and primary care physicians (see figure 1-A). Thus, even though psychiatrists represent the branch of medicine that specializes in psychopharmacology, they are directly responsible for providing only a fraction of professional services to the mentally ill. Consequently, it is becoming increasingly important for all mental health clinicians to have a basic familiarity with psychiatric medication treatment.

Many nonmedical psychotherapists are or will become strongly and rather directly involved in medication treatment. In some settings psychologists and social workers assume a major role in monitoring client responses to psychotropic medications. As primary therapist, these practitioners are in most frequent contact with clients and are in the best position to observe symptomatic improvement, side effect problems, and issues involving medication compliance. When consulting with primary care physicians, or as a staff member in some HMO settings, nonmedical therapists who are well-versed in the use of psychiatric medications can play an active (albeit collaborative) role in recommending particular medications and dosage adjustments. In addition, the Department of Defense, in response to an inadequate number of psychiatrists available in the military, has recently implemented a pilot program to train a small number of psychologists so that they are able to prescribe a limited formulary of psychiatric medications. These various activities reflect quite direct involvement in medication treatment by nonmedical therapists.

Who Writes Prescriptions for Psychotropic Medications

Class of Medications	Psychiatrists (%)	Nonpsychiatric M.D.s (%)
Antipsychotics	40	60
Antidepressants	31	69
Antianxiety	10	90
Hypnotics	11	89
Lithium	62	38

Source: Beardsley et al. 1988

Figure 1-A

In contrast, many nonmedical therapists have little to do with drug treatment. In some cases this may be due to the nature of their position in a particular treatment setting, in others it may have more to do with their own preferences and biases, such as opposition to medication treatment. However, we believe that, regardless of the degree of involvement and interest in medication treatment, it is increasingly important that *all* mental health therapists become acquainted with some basic notions regarding psychopharmacology.

Convincing evidence now exists that certain mental disorders are either caused by or accompanied by neurochemical abnormalities. The failure to appropriately diagnose and medically treat such conditions can result in the use of ineffective or only partially effective treatments and hence in prolonged suffering. Aside from the obvious cost in human terms, prolonged inappropriate treatment results in excessive financial burdens for clients, their families, and the health care system.

In addition, to date there have been successful malpractice suits brought against therapists who failed to treat or refer for treatment patients suffering from particular disorders known to be generally responsive to medication.

All mental health professionals must be able to, at the very least, diagnose mental disorders that require psychotropic medication treatment so that appropriate referrals can be made. Differential diagnosis will be discussed in detail in this book.

In many cases, clients may not choose to see a psychiatrist, even when told by their therapist that medication treatment is indicated. This may be due to financial concerns or to the negative stigma some people believe is attached to psychiatric treatment. A viable alternative, in some cases, is referral to the family practice doctor. Many people suffering from emotional distress see their family physician first. This doctor may begin treatment with psychotropic medications and may also refer the patient for psychotherapy. In such cases, the nonmedical therapist may be in a key position to supply information regarding diagnosis and treatment response. Increasingly, family practice physicians and nonmedical therapists become partners collaborating on the treatment of many clients—especially those suffering from fairly uncomplicated depressive and anxiety disorders.

Effective consultation with family practice doctors and psychiatrists alike is enhanced by the nonmedical therapist's ability to accurately communicate and discuss diagnosis, target symptoms, presumed etiology, and possible treatments. We are hopeful that this book will provide a solid grounding in basic issues to help improve communication and cooperation between professionals.

Mental health treatment has moved increasingly toward greater acceptance of multidisciplinary and integrated treatment modalities. As sophistication in the diagnosis and medical treatment of mental disorders continues to develop, it will be important that mental health professionals not take a step backward. The polarization of models and professional "turf battles" of the sixties and seventies may have sparked useful and lively debate, but they also often resulted in a fragmentation of care. Ongoing knowledge of and respect for diverse models and collaborative involvement hold promise for increasingly effective efforts in treating mental illness.

2

Integrated Models

The decision about whether to use psychotropic medications in the treatment of psychiatric disorders is influenced by a number of factors. Unfortunately, often the decision is based largely on the clinician's a priori view toward treatment, deriving from his or her theoretical perspective. As we shall argue, the critical variable in this decision is more appropriately based on the diagnosis, and in particular on the presence or absence of key target symptoms that suggest the patient is experiencing some form of neurochemical disorder.

In broad and extremely heterogeneous groups of disorders, such as mood disorders, *some* may be largely or exclusively caused by biological factors. Other disorders in such groups share *some* symptoms with biologic-based mental illness, yet their etiology stems largely or exclusively from nonbiologic sources, for example, emotional, psychosocial, or cognitive sources. Thus a very important question to address when making a diagnosis and subsequent decisions about treatment is, "Is there any evidence to suggest that this person's problems are due to some form of biologic disturbance?" However, all too often this question is framed overly simplistically: "Is the disorder biological or is it psychological?"

The distinction between what is psyche and what is soma is ambiguous at best. Invariably, there is a complex interaction between psychological and biological factors in all cases of emotional disorder. This complexity will be the focus of this chapter.

Psychology and Biology: A Two-Way Street

A comprehensive discussion of the classic, philosophical issue, mind-brain dualism, is beyond the scope of this book. (The reader is referred to Goodman 1991; Young

1987.) However, we would like to highlight a small number of cases and research studies that illustrate the interactive effects of biologic and psychologic factors.

Biological Factors, Impact on Psychological Functioning

> Men ought to know that from the brain, and from the brain only, arise our pleasures, joys, laughter, and jests, as well as our sorrows, pains, griefs, and fears ... It is the same thing which makes us mad or delirious, inspires us with dread and fear, whether by night or by day, brings sleeplessness, inopportune mistakes, aimless anxieties, absentmindedness, and acts that are contrary to habit.
>
> —Hippocrates

For the past two thousand plus years, there has been at least rudimentary recognition of the brain as the site of reasoning and emotions.

Early physicians were keen to note that brain injuries could result in profound changes in personality, cognition, and emotional control. And, as noted in chapter 1, in the earliest days of modern psychiatry the field was grounded in biological sciences and the medical model.

Two fairly common clinical examples serve as illustrations of how disordered brain functioning can lead to marked psychiatric symptomatology.

Case 1

Robert B. is a 42-year-old stockbroker. He has always been an ambitious, bright, energetic man. Despite normal stresses of daily life, he never experienced major psychiatric problems until a month ago. For no apparent reason he began gradually to slip into a state of lethargy, fatigue, and low motivation. His normal zest for life diminished, his usual sharpness of wit became dull, and his sense of enthusiasm gave way to increasing blandness and emptiness. He was totally perplexed as he searched his recent life experiences to find the cause for his malady. None was to be found.

In the ensuing weeks he lost weight, frequently woke at 3:00 AM and was unable to go back to sleep, and lost all sexual desire for his wife.

Upon close investigation by his family physician, it was eventually discovered that the depressive symptoms began several weeks after he had started taking an antihypertensive drug to treat his high blood pressure. The medication was suspect and was eventually changed. Within a couple of weeks, the depression vanished.

This case illustrates how a medication can, at times, dramatically alter a person's brain chemistry, resulting in major psychiatric symptoms. In Robert's case, there was no evidence of long-standing psychological problems and no clear psychological stressors.

The brain can be seen, in a sense, as a tremendously complex biological ecosystem. As in other ecosystems, global functioning and survival depends on a large number of interrelated variables. At times, small changes in one aspect of the system influence a number of other variables—in essence, sending a ripple effect throughout the entire system. In the brain, often certain delicately balanced neurochemical systems can be altered (the term often used is *dysregulated*), resulting in a cascade of alterations affecting many other neurochemicals and the functioning of a host of brain structures. A drug, as in the example above, is but one of many variables that can result in neurochemical dysregulation and resulting psychiatric symptoms. (More will be said about other causes later in the chapter.)

Case 2

Elizabeth M. is a 68-year-old retired accountant whose passion is gardening. However, during the past three months she became unable to tend her garden for more than a few minutes at a time. She was almost constantly seized by tremendous restlessness and agitation, fretting, wringing her hands, and pacing about her house. "I feel like I am going to crawl out of my skin," she said.

Elizabeth lost 25 pounds over this three-month period and suffered fitful sleep. She also began to contemplate suicide. Her hopes for a well-deserved, peaceful retirement seemed to have been erased, as if she were plagued by some kind of curse. She could pinpoint absolutely no painful life events that might give meaning to her condition.

Fortunately, ultimately it was discovered that she was suffering from hyperthyroidism. Following successful treatment, she has been able to return to her garden and her life.

In this case, a metabolic disorder was the culprit. In the cases of both Robert and Elizabeth, neurochemical and hormonal factors grossly interfered with brain functioning. In both cases, the people were radically changed. Their perceptions were altered (pessimism, hopelessness), their sense of self was shaken, their emotions were out of control, and their physiological functioning had been derailed. Certainly they had strong emotional reactions to these changes (a phenomenon sometimes referred to as secondary emotional symptoms), however, in both cases the *primary* etiology was biological.

All mental health clinicians will encounter clients who present for treatment with presumed psychological problems but who in fact are suffering from biologically based disorders. Such disorders fall into three categories:

- Due to medical illnesses (such as hyperthyroidism)

- Due to drugs (prescribed, over-the-counter, or recreational)

- Endogenous mental illnesses [1]

---

1. The term *endogenous* means "arises from within." Certain psychiatric disorders have been found to be largely endogenous; that is, they arise spontaneously in the absence of provoking psychosocial stressors. The disorders can be attributed to a biological abnormality or a predisposition or vulnerability to dysfunction. Many of the so-called endogenous disorders appear to carry a *genetic loading*: are passed from generation to generation and presumably can be linked to certain genetic factors. More will be said about endogenous psychiatric disorders in subsequent chapters.

Psychological Factors' Impact on Biological Functioning

For a very long time there has been some vague notion that emotional stress can affect physiology. For example, for hundreds of years it has been noted that severe stress can lead to disease. Family physicians have long noted that in the wake of tragic losses, the bereaved easily fall prey to illness. Yet not until this century did the psychology-biology interaction begin to be explored. Psychosomatic medicine was ushered in by the pioneering work of Franz Alexander in the 1940s. And an explosion of interest and research has been seen in the eighties and nineties in the emerging field of psycho-neuro-immunology—the study of the effects of emotional factors on disease susceptibility and disease resistance.

It would require several textbooks to even begin to review the literature in psychosomatics and psycho-neuro-immunology. We would, however, like to briefly discuss a few studies that shed some light on the issue of the interaction of psychology and biology and its relationship to mental illnesses. The first two of these studies involved experimentation with animals.

• E. Kandel and colleagues have studied the effects of environmental experiences and learning on the nervous system in the *Aplysia* (a marine mollusk). This animal is well suited for such a study because its nerve cells are quite large and easy to visualize. Also it does respond well to learning experiments such as habituation, sensitization, and classical conditioning (Pinsker et al. 1970).

The researchers were able to trace neural pathways from touch receptors in the mollusk's gill and siphon, through its primitive nervous system, and out into corresponding motor neurons. Using repeated exposures to mild aversive stimuli, the investigators were able to document specific biochemical changes at the synapse, as well as structural changes in specific nerve cells. Conclusion: Environmental events and learning are actually accompanied by measurable changes in nerve cells; the animal's biology is altered.

• Neurologic changes have similarly been demonstrated in studies of learned helplessness in rats. In these classic studies, animals are exposed to extremely aversive conditions, from which they have no escape. After a period of exposure, the animals begin to exhibit marked behavioral changes: They become passive and immobile. And they fail to mount coping responses (escape) from later aversive situations from which escape *is* possible. In many respects, the animals have learned that they are helpless to respond, then they come to take on characteristics that resemble major depression in humans. Interestingly, not only do these helpless rats behave in a depressed manner, but their biochemical functioning is altered. Measures of brain chemistry reveal neurochemical alterations that are identical to those seen in humans suffering from severe grief reactions or clinical depression. Again, environmental experiences have modified brain functioning (Weiss, Glazer, and Pohorecky 1976).

• In very similar ways, in numerous studies the biochemistry of people with reactive depressions has been shown to be markedly altered. For example, emotionally healthy individuals without a personal or family history of depression who encounter major psychosocial stressors (especially losses) often become depressed. Presumably such people are not especially at risk (biologically or psychologically) for depression, but nonetheless they become depressed in response to significant stressful events. Further, in the course of their reaction, *some* patients develop not only emotional symptoms (sadness, pessimism, low self-esteem) but also a host of biologic symptoms, such as sleep disturbances, and marked biochemical abnormalities. The chemical dysfunctions include dysregulation of both neurotransmitters in the brain and hormones (for instance, adrenal hormones such as cortisol). Metabolic by-products of neurotransmitters have been measured indirectly in assays of spinal fluid, blood, and urine and by way of brain-imaging techniques such as PET and SPECT scanning.

  • Baxter et al. (1992) have convincingly demonstrated that psychotherapy can affect brain functioning. PET scans allow researchers to directly image living brain tissue and thus provide data on metabolic activity of specific areas of the brain. Studies using PET scans in severe obsessive-compulsive disorder reveal a localized brain abnormality: a metabolic disturbance in the head of the candate nucleus, a brain structure that is part of the basal ganglia. In obsessive-compulsive disorder, when individuals are symptomatic this abnormality is visible on PET scans. Yet following successful *behavioral* treatment (exposure and response-prevention treatments) the functioning of this brain area normalizes.

  • Evidence also exists supporting the theory that the earliest episodes of affective illnesses in bipolar patients are often "reactive" in nature; that is, the initial episode is not an endogenous, biologic event but rather is evoked by psychological stressors. As a consequence of the initial episode, neurons in key areas of the limbic system may undergo a process of modification (neurochemically and even structurally), whereby the brain is changed more or less permanently. The result of this is that, following the first one or two episodes, the altered brain functioning leaves the nervous system at much greater risk for subsequent episodes and sets in motion an endogenous process whereby affective episodes can occur spontaneously, even in the absence of psychological stress. From that point on, if the disorder is not controlled, each episode further affects the nervous system; the threshold for recurring episodes becomes progressively lower. This process is known as *kindling*. It begins as a response to external stressors and evolves into a largely biological illness.

These are but a few of many studies and clinical findings that collectively provide strong support for the idea that environmental and psychological factors can significantly affect biologic and neurologic functioning.

Biological-Psychological Interactions

It is very likely that complex, interactive effects exist between biological and psychological factors. It's never a question of all or none. In the case of Robert B., he was suffering from an endogenous depression and experiencing marked lethargy, poor concentration, and low motivation. This eventually lead to performance problems at work, and a number of critical remarks from his boss. These events began to fuel the flame of low self-esteem. Low self-esteem is generally not felt to be a primary symptom of biologically based depressive disorders, but it is almost universally seen to emerge as patients live with ongoing clinical depression.

Biologic effects may secondarily affect psychological functioning in a number of ways, among them:

  • Altered perception. Biologic effects can contribute to the pessimistic thinking seen in depressive disorders and the tendency to anticipate fearful outcomes often seen in anxiety disorders.

- Increased emotional sensitivity and reduced emotional controls. Increased emotional arousal or pain may motivate a person to become more socially withdrawn and can often lead to a host of negative conclusions regarding personal competency, as in, "What's wrong with me? I'm crying like a baby."

- Decreased energy and arousal, poor concentration, and lowered motivation, which often leads to impaired performance in school and work.

- Sexual dysfunction, which can translate into interpersonal problems in intimate relationships.

- Bizarre behavior enacted during a psychotic episode. Such behavior can continue to be a source of tremendous personal embarrassment and shame long after the psychotic episode is resolved.

These consequences of a primarily biologically based mental disorder have an impact on the individual's sense of self-worth and competency in the world. Conversely, this increased level of despair can, in itself, operate to intensify the underlying biological abnormality.

Practical Implications

As previously mentioned, the question "Is this disorder psychological or is it biological?" is too simplistic. The more appropriate question is "To what extent is there evidence that biochemical factors may be contributing to a patient's current symptomatology?" This is much more than an academic question. To the extent that we can determine biologic etiology (or at least a degree of biologic dysfunction as a part of the more global disorder), pharmacologic treatments may be indicated. (How a biologic etiology and the need for medication are determined is addressed in detail in later chapters.)

Stimulus-Response Specificity

Stimulus-response specificity is a concept describing conditions where a very specific response can be predicted with tremendous regularity when a stimulus is applied. One example would be that an electrical shock to muscle tissue evokes a contraction. This model is appropriate for some types of medical interventions. For example, for acute cardiac and respiratory arrest, the techniques of cardiopulmonary resuscitation (CPR) can be used with most victims, regardless of their age, socioeconomic status, sex, or religious beliefs. When there is an obstructed airway, performing an emergency tracheotomy is appropriate for victims regardless of their emotional status, personality style, or level of psychosocial maturity. Likewise, some medications have fairly universal effects on all people; for instance, sodium pentothal produces unconsciousness (Deckert 1985).

Medical treatments in psychiatry generally *do not* follow the rule of stimulus-response specificity. Although the particular mechanism of drug action may be identified, the same medication given to two depressed patients, for example, may affect them very differently. Some of these differences may be traced to variations in metabolism from individual to individual (see chapter 3). Or the underlying biochemical abnormality in one depressed patient may be different than the abnormality in another depressed patient, and thus the medications affect different underlying disorders.

Beyond these physiological differences, however, the patients' responses may be influenced to a significant degree by a host of social, cognitive, and personality factors that have little or nothing to do with biology. In the realm of psychiatric medication treatment, socio-cultural experiences and beliefs, personality style, and a vast number of personal psychodynamic factors can, and do, dramatically influence patient response. Psychological functioning cannot be understood using the simple, reductionist notions implied in stimulus-response specificity.

The good clinician *always* treats the person, not just the disorder. We may choose to influence nerve cells with psychotropic drugs, but the response will always be woven into the complex fabric of highly idiosyncratic personality factors. Therefore, successful pharmacologic treatment *always* requires a thorough knowledge of, not only the diagnosis and pathology and the medications used, but the unique meaning of the treatment to the individual patient. Assembly-line psychotropic treatment often fails, not because medications are ineffective, but because clinicians do not take time to understand their patients.

Unfortunately, in many overcrowded mental health clinics, some clinicians act as if stimulus-response specificity is appropriate. The result is that often these attempts at treatment efficiency and cost containment backfire. Many patients don't respond well and either must demand further outpatient services or continue to decompensate until they require hospitalization. And, of course, there is the human cost associated with prolonged suffering.

In the remainder of the chapter, we explore a number of ideas regarding psychological factors that have direct bearing on the outcome of medication treatment.

The Psychodynamics of Pharmacologic Treatment

When a prescription is written and a pill is taken, the effects of the medication are almost always influenced by a number of psychological factors. Some of these factors have to do with the commonly held beliefs regarding "drugs" and "illness" that are etched into the experience of most people in our culture. Other factors spring from highly personal, idiosyncratic sources, either in conscious awareness or buried deeply in the unconscious mind.

The astute clinician should continually ask the questions "If medications are suggested or prescribed, how will this be perceived by my patient?" and "What personal meaning might be attached to this form of intervention?" Prescribing and recommending medication always occurs in an interpersonal context. It is not like a landscaper recommending and applying a particular fertilizer to your lawn. Rather, it can be a highly personalized communication between therapist and client, a communication ripe for all sorts of transference distortions and a type of interaction that *may* alter the nature of the therapeutic relationship.

In addressing these issues, we will first speak about rather common, generic themes, and then go on to describe more unique, personal concerns. Let's consider some of the possible consequences.

Generic Meanings

In our culture, certain themes are evident in our cliches and language that link the taking of medicine with badness and punishment. The saying "Give him a taste of his own medicine" is but one example. One of the classic scenes from the *"Our Gang"* movie shorts has the wicked stepmother punishing Spanky and Alfalfa by making them swallow castor oil. Hearing bad news or carrying out unpleasant tasks is sometimes referred to as having to "swallow a bitter pill." Even in mature adults these connections between "taking your medicine" and punishment may echo at unconscious levels.

Probably more common are notions regarding medication and "being sick." Many psychiatric patients may be able to view their difficulties honorably, as "problems in living," and yet feel shamed and humiliated by a suggestion that they take psychotropic medications. The unspoken meaning they perceive may be "You need medications, thus you are *sick*." And being sick, in psychological terms, often carries its own assortment of negative connotations: weak, inadequate, crazy, deranged, and so on.

A common underlying concern sparked by the recommendation for psychotropics is "The therapist must think I can't handle things on my own—thinks I need a crutch." This can not only be wounding to the client's self-image, but may undermine the client's belief that the therapist is hopeful regarding his or her capacity for growth and healing.

Morality pervades many beliefs about the taking of drugs for emotional problems. Some people erroneously assume that all psychiatric drugs are alike. They conclude that all psychotropics are "tranquilizers," that all can lead to drug addiction, and that such dependence on drugs is little different than alcoholism. Thus, if you take drugs, you are bad, or at the very least, weak willed. This view of drugs as evil, or at least as dangerously addictive, is often adopted by twelve-step chemical dependency programs. The lay leaders of some twelve-step groups are understandably skeptical and afraid of drugs that can lead to abuse, but may be ignorant of the fact that most psychotropic medications are not addictive at all. It is all too common for someone who has received a dual diagnosis of, for example alcohol abuse and major depression, to encounter tremendous pressure in his or her twelve-step recovery program to discontinue antidepressant medication. Fortunately, many recovery programs are learning about the appropriate use of some psychiatric medications, and understand their role in treating dual-diagnosis clients.

Finally, psychiatric drugs are seen by some as an assault on free will and autonomy. Certainly this idea has been brought to our attention by media reports of instances in which psychotropic drugs have been used solely to achieve behavioral control. "Chemical straitjackets" and other forms of biological restraint, such as lobotomies, have been the subject of popular film and television productions (for example *One Flew Over the Cuckoo's Nest, Frances*, and *Will There Really Be a Morning?*). And clearly these abuses have and do occur. However, appropriately used medical interventions oftentimes work to free people and promote autonomy.

Case 3

Sara M. is a 34-year-old housewife. Over the past two years she has been plagued by devastating panic attacks and unable to leave her home or to be alone. Her husband must have relatives stay with Sara or hire a "babysitter" to be with her when he goes to work. Sara is frightened, and she feels humiliated.

Sara initially balked at the suggestion that she take psychiatric medications. She saw the recommendation as an attack on her sense of adequacy and worth. However, after a period of psychotherapy, she did agree to take the medications. After eight weeks of treatment with imipramine and clonazepam she was free from panic attacks and began to venture out of her home for the first time in two years. Six months later she was reentering the mainstream of life and had just attended a performance of the local symphony. One of her greatest personal losses had been her inability to attend the symphony.

For Sara, the medication played a key role in reducing panic symptoms. But it was her own courage that enabled her to resume normal living, as she gradually chose to go outside her home or to spend time alone. In Sara's case, medications played *a part* in restoring her autonomy and bringing her back to life.

Case 4

One of the authors treated a young woman, Ellen G., who came for her first appointment at the mental health clinic with this opening line: "I'm starting to fall apart again. I guessed it was time to come in and start taking my Thorazine again." She had been treated with this antipsychotic drug off and on for the past three years and was now consulting with a new therapist. The therapist commented, "Well, maybe you're right about needing the medication again. But let's take some time to talk and see if we can understand what's going on for you."

As her story unfolded, it became clear that she was experiencing symptoms of a serious, delayed-onset post-traumatic stress disorder. In prior treatments, her therapists had never explored her circumstances beyond observing her feelings of panic, depersonalization, and confusion. They were quick to medicate her and seal over her distress.

In the current treatment, medications were not used. Months later this woman remarked, "That first day when you didn't just give me meds, but said 'Let's talk' ... It was the first time I started to feel hopeful about therapy."

When medications are given, especially if they are offered or recommended early on in treatment, many clients' perception is "They just want to drug me. They don't want to talk ... They don't want to hear my pain." Patients may feel they are being treated as a "case" (as in stimulus-response specificity) and the result can be a serious warp in the developing therapeutic alliance or even premature termination of therapy.

At times when therapists feel stuck with a client, their own sense of futility or impotence may lead to the decision to try medications. This feeling of pessimism may be picked up on by the client. As Jerome Frank (1973) and others have argued, one of the most important roles therapists can play is to help maintain realistic hopefulness, especially during times when clients are feeling especially demoralized. Certainly, psychotropic medications may be indicated and can be crucial interventions with *some* "stuck" psychotherapy clients. However, the choice to medicate should be based on thorough consideration of diagnostic issues, and not be simply a response to the therapist's own pessimism.

Personal Meanings

Just like any other type of intervention or communication in therapy, the therapist's behaviors and interactions can certainly be perceived in particular, unique ways by the client—ways that make sense when the client's psychodynamics are understood. Although such personal dynamics vary tremendously from person to person, we would like to address several fairly common examples that can be seen in clinical practice.

Dependent patients

The request for medications (explicit or implicit) by dependent patients, often conveys a need to be fed. Aside from direct medication effects, the gratification experienced by the patient when given drugs may account for symptomatic improvement. It is also important to note that once the therapist prescribes medications (however appropriate this may be) in some way he or she has strayed from a position of neutrality, and this may have consequences for the therapeutic relationship. Conversely, the choice not to prescribe or recommend medications may be seen as "withholding." The symbolic-dynamic issues discussed here are also important concerns in the treatment of clients with borderline personality disorders.

Obsessive-compulsive patients

People with obsessive-compulsive personality styles value control and precise intellectual scrutiny. Thus, when medications are prescribed, the therapist will often be confronted with (1) a request for detailed information about the medication and its side effects, (2) frequent discussions regarding medication response and side effects (even *very* minor side effect problems), and (3) worries centering around loss of control experiences that may result from even very minimal side effects, such as slight degree of sedation or dizziness.

Case 5

Albert K. is a 54-year-old engineer, receiving treatment for a major depression. This rigid, obsessional man came for his appointment a week after being started on tricyclic antidepressants. During the past week he had written a computer program to track medication side effects on a daily basis, and he brought a data sheet with him to the session. The program addressed fifteen different side effects (which he had gleaned from the *Physicians' Desk Reference*); each one was rated daily on a scale of 1 to 10, and results were displayed in terms of daily scores and weekly averages and on bar graphs. This was Albert's style, his way of approaching medication treatment. The therapist thought it was a classic for obsessional patients and was impressed with Albert's program and charts.

Anxious patients

Individuals who suffer from severe anxiety disorders and, in particular, phobias and panic disorder, already experience a significant amount of fearfulness in their daily life. Oftentimes when medications are prescribed, the medication itself becomes a new source of fear for these patients. This is frequently seen when such individuals are started on antidepressant medications. These medications may present some side effects, such as a rapid heart rate, and these are quickly interpreted by the anxious patient as a sign of increased anxiety and loss of control. This may lead to patients' quickly discontinuing the medication or even therapy itself.

Paranoid patients

The issues encountered with paranoid patients often surround struggles over control and autonomy. These people are especially frightened by others assuming a position of control over them, and being "medicated" often touches on this theme. In more-psychotic paranoid patients, this issue not uncommonly takes the form of delusions in which the patient feels the therapist is trying to poison him or her.

Depressed patients

Frequently, seriously depressed patients, when encountering very minor side effect problems, complain bitterly about these difficulties or abruptly discontinue antidepressant medication treatment. It may be difficult to understand why a morbidly depressed person would abandon treatment when all he or she has encountered is a slightly dry mouth or minor degree of sedation. Yet it bears keeping in mind that such people are already exquisitely sensitive to discomfort, overwhelmed by psychological pain, and prone to tremendous pessimism. Although the therapist hopes for significant benefit from the antidepressant, the patient's experience is often focused on a here-and-now awareness of added discomfort and probably persistently bleak view of the future.

Narcissistic patients

The never-ending search for the perfect relationship, the perfect job, and the perfect life that narcissistic patients pursue may extend to the demand for the perfect medication—which pharmaceutical companies have not as yet developed.

Medication as a tool for resistance

Across diagnostic groups, a common experience is for the patient to bring up medication and medication problems as a form of resistance. It is of course, important to track medication responses and encourage patient-therapist dialogue regarding effects. However, when this topic comes to dominate too much of the therapy hour, it may be an indication that the subject is being used in the service of resistance. That is, the focus is shifted away from inner thoughts and feelings to symptoms and side effects. In addition, arguments or complaints regarding medication issues may also become an arena for struggles over control.

Countertransference issues

Medications are sometimes given to patients in a sort of "rescue response," when the therapist either fears the therapy is ineffective or worried about the patient experiencing excessive emotional pain. Although certainly this may be appropriate at times, it can also be a countertransference problem that interferes with treatment.

A therapist will sometimes give medications to a patient to soften the blow of termination or to assuage the therapist's guilt over stopping treatment—a problem seen more commonly these days in short-term therapy clinics. Some clinics offer only limited psychotherapy, but will allow patients to continue some form of contact with therapists if they are on medications. So prescribing medications can be a way to "legitimize" continued contact and avoid the losses associated with termination.

It is not our goal to recommend specific solutions to these various client dynamics or countertransference problems but rather to highlight them as particular concerns. The well-trained therapist never views medication treatment in a vacuum or as a stimulus-response specific intervention. Alertness to these issues and a willingness to inquire about personal interpretation of the recommendation for medication are our best hedge against problems that can potentially derail treatment or contribute to poor medication compliance.

3

Pharmacology and Neurophysiology

Psychiatry, perhaps uniquely in health care, operates from an established multidisciplinary approach. The opportunity, as well as the responsibility, exists for all clinicians to be involved in medication decisions as appropriate to their discipline. As treatment approaches in mental health continue to evolve, it is likely that current practices will expand and demand participation from knowledgeable therapists.

From a practical standpoint, possessing fundamental knowledge is critical in the rapidly changing field of psychopharmacology, along with the attendant challenge of understanding emerging treatments, new applications of existing medications, and multiple drug regimens. Additionally, medical comorbidity in psychiatric patients (coexisting medical illness and psychiatric disorder) mandates at least a familiarity with psychotropics' potential actions and interactions with various non-psychotropic therapeutic agents.

In your practice as a nonmedical psychotherapist, it is not essential to become an expert in the area of physiology, pharmacology, or biochemistry. However, it is important to become generally familiar with a few preliminary concepts, which will lay a groundwork for the clinical chapters which follow. This chapter presents basic pharmacologic principles, defines terminologies commonly found in later chapters of this book (and in standard medical or medication texts), and integrates factual information about neurophysiology and brain functioning.

Basic Principles of Pharmacokinetics

The broad definition of a drug as "any chemical that affects living processes" (Benet, Mitchell, and Sherner 1990a) is helpful in understanding the relationship between the body and administered medications. This is a fluid and interactive process, composed of two elements: *pharmacodynamics* and *pharmacokinetics*.

Pharmacodynamics can be viewed as the drug's effect on the body (discussed in detail for specific drugs in part three of this book). Conversely, pharmacokinetics can be considered the body's effect on the drug. There are four basic pharmacokinetic factors: *absorption, distribution, biotransformation,* and *excretion* (see figure 3-A). Every drug will exhibit a unique kinetic profile (like a fingerprint) composed of these factors. This chapter provides a general description of pharmacokinetic principles and their significance in clinical practice. (Expanded discussion for each area of pharmacokinetics is provided in appendix A.)

Absorption

Most drugs are initially, and predominantly, absorbed in the stomach or small intestine. The degree of absorption in the digestive tract can be affected by patient-dependent factors, such as whether the medication is taken with or without food. Further, as a drug proceeds to its ultimate destination, it may have numerous barriers to cross, depending on the absorption characteristics of the drug itself. For instance, in the central nervous system (CNS), the blood-brain barrier allows passage of only certain molecules into the brain. Penetration of medication into the CNS is restricted by a host of factors which protect the CNS from exposure to toxins, although this is not absolute or impenetrable. (See appendix A for discussion of related factors of bioavailability and first-pass phenomena.)

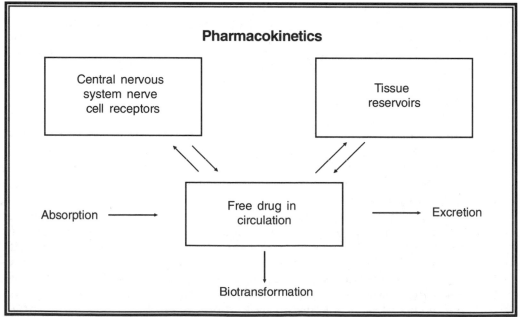

Figure 3-A

Case 6

Patricia A. is a 45-year-old female referred to the day treatment program at your hospital. She is an intelligent, energetic woman whose chief complaint is "difficulty remembering things." She is moderately anxious about this symptom, since she is expecting to return to work in two weeks after a six-month medical leave of absence. She was diagnosed with breast cancer seven months ago, for which she received chemotherapy and radiation treatment. Tests indicate that her cancer has not spread, and her physician reports an excellent prognosis.

Patricia is a member of a support group for cancer survivors which has helped her "tremendously." She is hoping someone in your program can help her "get a handle on this memory thing." Her job requires that she retain and recall detailed numerical data, and she does not want to return to work "less than 100 percent." You will be providing psychotherapy to her on a daily basis for the next ten days.

During your initial session with her, she tells you that she is sure that her memory loss is related to the effects of her chemotherapy and is therefore somewhat doubtful that you will be able to help her. You find that this might be a reasonable question to pursue before proceeding too far in therapy with her. Your program relies heavily on interdisciplinary treatment, so you request psychological testing from the psychologist and a medication review from the pharmacist. Psychological testing results show Patricia to be above average in intelligence with no evidence of organicity or personality disorder. The pharmacist reports that none of the chemotherapeutic agents that Patricia received crosses the blood-brain barrier appreciably or affects healthy brain tissue.

Typical memory loss secondary to cancer treatment is short term and is usually attributable to pretreatment antianxiety medications. Based on these reports, you feel confident in moving ahead with therapy and exploring Patricia's anxiety and memory loss from a nonorganic focus.

Distribution

Once a drug has been absorbed and reaches the bloodstream, it is then distributed to various organs or sites of action throughout the body. Certain medications have characteristic distribution patterns, which are extremely important in understanding response to treatment. A critical example in psychiatry is the extensive depositing of tricyclic antidepressants and antipsychotic medications in fat and muscle cells. In effect, these areas act as reservoirs or holding tanks. In some instances, concentrations of a drug in reservoir areas will exceed levels in the bloodstream. This explains why serum levels of antidepressants are not absolutely indicative of total body concentration. (See appendix A for a detailed description of distribution phases and protein binding.)

Case 7

Helen P. is an obese 27-year-old woman who has been taking the antidepressant desipramine. She was started on a low dose and gradually increased to a dose of 300 mg daily, which she has been taking for the past three months. Even though Helen has only in the last two months been able to notice an effect, she now reports a significant improvement in her depression and no side effects. Her physician has forwarded results of periodic desipramine blood levels to you, and all are within therapeutic range. However, Helen recently discovered that a coworker also takes this medication, in a dose of 150 mg daily, and is doing well. She reveals to you that without consulting her physician she has cut her dose in half over the last two weeks because she thinks her dosage was too high.

You firmly encourage Helen to discuss this matter with her doctor, and point out to her that a dose of 300 mg is still within the standard accepted dosage range and that blood level monitoring has shown this dose to be right for her. You further remind her of the risk and consequences if her depression should recur. Because you are aware that this tricyclic antidepressant is probably extensively stored in her fat tissue you are able to provide needed reassurance that her treatment is reasonable and being safely monitored.

Biotransformation

The body's reaction to drugs as foreign substances results in several processes of elimination, one being metabolism (biotransformation) and the other excretion. Metabolism occurs primarily in the liver, via specific action of enzymes that change the original chemical into compounds that are more easily excreted by the kidneys. Biotransformation is a complex process. Understanding metabolic activity is crucial in medication management, especially when medication treatment is not working adequately.

When medications are chemically altered by the process of biotransformation, the results are the production of numerous chemical by-products, called *metabolites*. Some metabolites are useful and desirable, in that they produce desired effects; for instance, the reduction of psychiatric symptoms. Unfortunately, some metabolites affect various bodily tissues and result in undesirable side effects. In addition, since most medications undergo significant metabolism, the risks of drug *toxicity* (poisoning due to excessively high levels of a drug) must be considered whenever metabolism is impaired. Antidepressants, antipsychotics, and anticonvulsants are all extensively metabolized by liver enzymes. Thus, impaired liver functioning can result in abnormal metabolism of these medications. Conversely, increased activity of liver enzymes can cause excessive metabolism, resulting in a decreased drug level and an inadequate response to treatment. (Appendix A contains additional information regarding metabolic enzymes and drug metabolites.)

Case 8

Harry Y. is a 50-year-old Asian man who has been referred to you for short-term therapy following a seven-day hospitalization for psychotic depression. He is currently taking an antidepressant, nortriptyline, at 75 mg daily, and a low-dose antipsychotic, thiothixene, at 4 mg daily, both at bedtime. Harry has no previous psychiatric history but states that he wants to "get better" and will take his medications as prescribed and do "whatever else you decide I need."

His initial psychotic symptoms were of a paranoid nature regarding his boss, but by Harry's report, "Those bad thoughts have gone away." He reports feeling less depressed than when admitted to the hospital but is still not "back to normal." Your initial impression is that Harry is committed to treatment, although you are bothered by his presentation, including marked drowsiness, slight hand tremor, periodic restlessness, and his description of extreme dry mouth. He describes being aware of all these signs but says that he was told the medications could cause such things and doesn't want to "bother his doctor."

Although you see many patients on meds, Harry's side effects seem extreme, and you place a call to his physician later in the day. She is appreciative of your call and agrees with your concerns. She decides to lower Harry's nortriptyline dose until she receives pending lab results of his nortriptyline level. She also shares with you information that indicates certain Asian populations may be unable to effectively metabolize tricyclic antidepressants and antipsychotics, necessitating lower than average doses. She promises to call you after further evaluation (Shimoda et al. 1993).

Excretion

Excretion is the process by which drugs are eliminated from the body. Excretion occurs primarily via the kidneys, although other routes include the gastrointestinal tract, the respiratory system, and sweat, saliva, and breast milk. Adequate excretion is dependent on effective kidney function. Disease- or drug-induced damage to the kidneys can lead to kidney failure, resulting in a toxic accumulation of medications in the bloodstream.

An important characteristic of medications is the *half-life* ($t_{1/2}$), which is defined as the amount of time required for the serum concentration to be reduced by 50 percent (Benet, Mitchell, and Sherner 1990b). Half-life is used to determine dosage amounts and intervals for most medications.

Half-life measurements are used to estimate the time required for a drug to reach what is called *steady state*. Steady state occurs when concentrations of a medication in the bloodstream have reached a plateau, so that the amount administered is equal to the amount being eliminated. It is generally accepted that for most drugs steady state is attained after four half-lives; for example if the half-life is 24 hours, then steady state is usually reached in four days. It is important to remember that reaching steady state does not always correspond to a drug's onset of desired action. With antidepressants, for instance, steady state will be reached long before a therapeutic effect is noted. (See figure 3-B; also see appendix A for discussion of a related topic, the therapeutic index.)

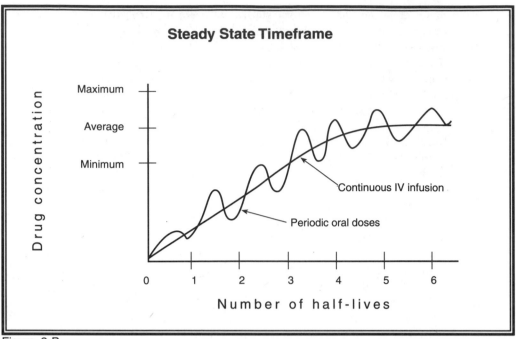

Figure 3-B

Case 9

Frank is a 24-year-old honor student, majoring in engineering, who you have been seeing for four months through the student counseling center. He initially presented with major depression, although he has never been suicidal. He has significant narcissistic and passive-aggressive traits. He began treatment with Prozac, 20 mg daily in the morning, two weeks ago. His agreement to take medications came after much discussion with you and the psychiatrist, including detailed information regarding dosage range, onset of action, and side effects.

During today's session, he angrily informs you that the medication is not working and challenges you to answer some questions he has formulated after reading the *Physicians' Desk Reference*. His opinion, based on mathematical calculations, is that the drug has had plenty of time to reach a therapeutic level. He concludes that "the whole idea is some sort of placebo experiment" and threatens to terminate treatment.

This behavior is characteristic of Frank, and you respond in a calm and nondefensive way. You acknowledge his need to thoroughly understand the medication and that it can be frustrating to wait for indicators that the drug is working. However, you remind him that the typical response time for most antidepressants is three to four weeks and is not absolutely related to serum level of the medication. You suggest other sources of information, written for patients, which may more specifically address his needs. You also offer encouragement that he has tolerated the medication without significant side effects.

Medication Effects

When medications are chemically reorganized into various metabolites, these resulting compounds produce a variety of effects—some desirable, some undesirable. All medications, including psychotropics, typically have five primary effects:

- *Pharmacological effect*—the desired therapeutic effect, such as antipsychotics reducing hallucinations.

- *Side effects*—typically considered to be undesirable effects, such as constipation, dry mouth, blurry vision, and so on. Occasionally side effects can be used to benefit the patient, for example, using a medication's sedating side effect to help an anxious patient fall asleep at night. Side effects, although generally undesirable, are by definition fairly common and predictable and may be somewhat preventable. Side effects are generally considered extensions of the pharmacological properties of a drug, and account for 70 to 80 percent of adverse drug events (Glazener 1992).

- *Idiosyncratic effects*—extremely rare, adverse effects, and are difficult to predict. They are often specific to an individual or to certain groups of patients who share common genetic or biologic features.

- *Allergic reactions*—some individuals have an immune response to medications, generally a skin rash or hypersensitivity. The body may respond to the medication as if it was a foreign substance or organism and produce allergic symptoms. A severe type of allergic reaction, called anaphylaxis, can include difficulty breathing, fever, and irregular heart beat. Anaphylactic reactions are potentially fatal, as is, for example, an allergy to penicillin.

- *Discontinuance syndrome*—response to stopping or interrupting medication treatment. Examples are narcotic withdrawal or "cholinergic rebound" when tricyclic antidepressants or antipsychotics are abruptly stopped.

Drug Interactions

Basic pharmacologic principles apply as much to drug *interactions* as to drug actions. Each kinetic property—absorption, distribution, metabolism (biotransformation), and excretion—is potentially affected by the presence of coadministered medications. Drug interactions follow a variable time-course pattern, from immediate to delayed. Consequently, it is important to remember that several weeks may elapse before the effects of an interactive combination are evident.

And the comorbidity of medical and psychiatric disorders requires at least some degree of multiple drug prescribing. For example, many patients suffering from serious physical disorders as well as depression will require medication treatment for both conditions. Examples include diabetes mellitus, cancer, and cardiovascular disease. Familiarity with drug interactions can be an important addition to diagnostic skills.

Although significant interactions for specific drugs will be addressed in subsequent chapters, case 10 illustrates the most frequently encountered of all drug interactions, enzyme inhibition (Hansten and Horn 1990). This interaction occurs when two drugs rely on the same enzyme system for metabolism. In this "competition," one drug usually wins over the other and is preferentially and completely metabolized. Conversely, metabolism of the other drug is inhibited, leading to an increased serum level. This increase can at times produce greater effectiveness than anticipated from a given dose, or it can produce serious adverse effects, such as toxicity.

Case 10

Gail F. is a 38-year-old female who has been in therapy with you for the last eight months. Her original presentation included significant vegetative symptoms of depression, including weight loss, insomnia, agitation, decreased libido, fatigue, and difficulty concentrating. After several sessions with you, she reluctantly agreed to see a psychiatrist in your group for medication evaluation. Even though she was hesitant to take meds, she indicated that she trusted your judgment and complied with the prescribed regimen of imipramine, slowly titrated (adjusted) to an eventual dose of 200 mg daily.

This therapy has proceeded relatively well in conjunction with continued psychotherapy working on issues surrounding sexual abuse she suffered as a child. She acknowledges a response to her antidepressant and having experienced minimal side effects of constipation and dry mouth in the first few weeks. However, in the session last week and again today she is complaining of "feeling dizzy" and of a "speeded-up heart rate." Additionally she describes the return of constipation and dry mouth similar to when she began imipramine. She insists upon focusing on these physical symptoms during the session and is pressuring you for advice on what to do. Upon inquiry, she reports that two weeks ago the physician for whom she works gave her a prescription for cimetidine to help with "ulcer pain." She has not informed this physician of her treatment with imipramine.

You refer Gail to the psychiatrist, who instructs her to discontinue imipramine and orders a blood level to be drawn that afternoon. The psychiatrist suspects that Gail's metabolism of imipramine may be impaired by the addition of cimetidine. The symptoms that Gail describes are consistent with tricyclic toxicity. Cimetidine is known to inhibit the ability of liver enzymes to metabolize numerous other medications, including antidepressants (American Society of Hospital Pharmacists 1993).

You find out several days later that Gail's imipramine level was elevated by about 40 percent. Her psychiatrist feels it will be safe for her to resume imipramine at a lower dose if she continues taking cimetidine. At her next session she is undecided about restarting her antidepressant and wishes to discuss it with you.

There is a likelihood that psychiatric patients (especially older people) will be receiving multiple medications. People with clinical syndromes that include associated physical symptoms, such as anxiety disorders and depression, are often initially treated by a nonpsychiatrist prescriber. The medications prescribed can include gastrointestinal agents, antihypertensives, analgesics, and sedative-hypnotics. Subsequent referral to a psychiatrist may result in the addition of a psychotropic medication. Thus the psychotherapist may ultimately inherit this patient with the attendant possibilities of drug interactions.

The presentation of this material does not suggest that psychotherapists are responsible for identifying and monitoring drug interactions. That is a job best left to physicians and pharmacists. However, in certain cases the effects of interactive drugs will be evident in therapy. For example, when a previously good medication response has abated, or when the intensity of side effects is inconsistent with dosage, ruling out drug interactions is helpful. Also, psychotherapists often have more complete information about a client's treatment than do individual physicians, each of whom may be independently prescribing potentially interactive medications. In these situations, it is the psychotherapist who often sounds the initial warning.

The Nervous System on a Cellular Level

The function of the nervous system depends on communication between nerve cells (*neurons*). Structurally, all neurons are composed of a *cell body, dendrites, axon*, and *terminal boutons* (see figure 3-C). Dendrites are short, terminally branched structures projecting out from the cell body. They receive and conduct information to the cell body; there may be one or several dendrites on each cell. Extremely fine projections on the dendrites are called *dendritic spines*. The axon is a single long fiber that ends in enlarged structures called terminal boutons. The axon serves to conduct impulses away from the cell body.

Neurons communicate unidirectionally. Information is received via the dendrite(s) and is passed through the cell body, along the axon, and out the bouton to the next neuron at a point of close proximity: the synapse. The majority of biologically based mental disorders can be traced to abnormalities in neuronal conduction at the synapse. Let's take a look at normal synaptic transmission and then see how this process can malfunction.

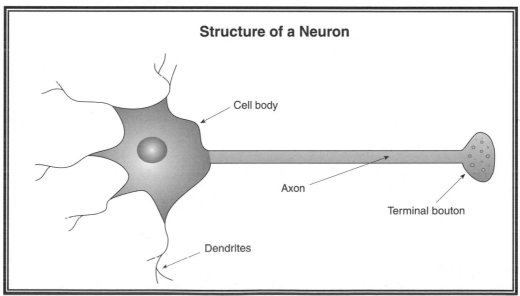

Structure of a Neuron

Cell body

Axon

Terminal bouton

Dendrites

Figure 3-C

Conduction and Transmission

The process of nerve activity begins with stimulation of the cell, resulting in a brief change in electrical potential from the cell's resting state. This change is termed an *action potential*. The action potential is converted into a nerve impulse as it spreads throughout the dendrites, cell body, and ultimately down the axon. At the nerve ending, the nerve impulse performs the critical function of causing the release of neurotransmitting chemicals into the synapse. The releasing side of the neuron is termed *presynaptic*. The process of impulse movement along the axon is termed *conduction; transmission* refers to passage of the impulse across the synaptic space (from one cell to the next).

Neurotransmitter chemicals are stored in small containers called vesicles, located inside the presynaptic terminal. Upon receiving stimulation from the action potential, the vesicles migrate toward the cell membrane, fuse with it, and discharge their contents into the synapse. On the adjacent, postsynaptic membrane are receptors (see figure 3-D).

Receptors are coiled proteins that weave in and out of the cell membrane. On the exterior surface of the receptor is a specialized area to which the neurotransmitter binds. When enough receptors are activated by the neurotransmitter, the nerve cell becomes activated and thus propagates the nerve impulse. *Neurotransmitters*, then, are chemical substances capable of binding to receptors, activating them, and resulting in the generation of an action potential—that is, in essence, they are capable of turning on the adjacent cell.

Neurotransmitters can be thought of as *first messengers*. The binding of a first messenger neurotransmitter may indirectly cause intracellular changes and activation of other chemicals *inside* the adjacent cell, which are called *secondary messengers*.

Most neurons are selective for the production and release of only one neurotransmitter. Neurotransmitters may elicit either an excitatory or an inhibitory action. The types and distribution of neurotransmitters are complex. (Figure 3-E shows the distribution of certain neurotransmitters in the brain.)

To date the following neurotransmitters have been identified: acetylcholine, norepinephrine, dopamine, glycine, serotonin (5-HT), gamma-aminobutyric acid (GABA), enkephalins, substance P, and glutamic acid.

In subsequent chapters the role of specific neurotransmitters in the etiology and treatment of psychiatric disorders will be explored.

Neuronal Malfunction

A number of things can go amiss in the process leading to a malfunction in neuronal firing. Let's take a look at several dysfunctions that underlie major mental illnesses (these abnormalities will be explored in greater detail in later chapters):

- The initial synthesis and production of the neurotransmitting chemical may be inhibited, thus little neurotransmitter is available for release.

- Certain biologically based disorders or drugs may either facilitate or inhibit the release of neurotransmitters by the presynaptic bouton.

- Nerve cells practice a sort of recycling, in which neurotransmitters already released are reabsorbed into the presynaptic cell; this process is referred to as *re-uptake* (see figure 3-D). Physiologic malfunctions and certain medications can either overstimulate or retard re-uptake.

- On the surface of pre- and postsynaptic cells are various types of inhibitory receptors. These receptors, rather than facilitating nerve firing, act as a brake

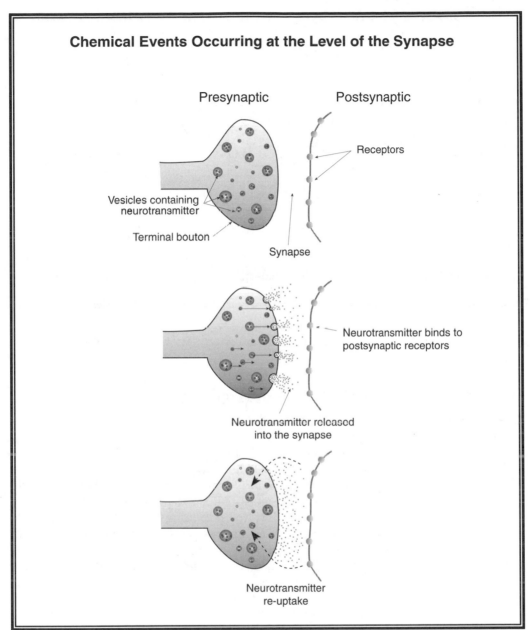

Chemical Events Occurring at the Level of the Synapse

Presynaptic

Postsynaptic

Receptors

Vesicles containing
neurotransmitter

Terminal bouton

Synapse

Neurotransmitter binds to
postsynaptic receptors

Neurotransmitter released
into the synapse

Neurotransmitter
re-uptake

Figure 3-D

and reduce the sensitivity of the nerve cell (make it less likely to fire). In certain conditions, the number of inhibitory receptors may actually increase (a process called *up-regulation*), which acts to decrease neuronal excitability. Conversely, in other conditions, the number of inhibitory receptors may become *down-regulated*, resulting in increased sensitivity.

- Finally, there is the process of neurotransmitter "waste management." Certain enzymes operate to biologically degrade neurotransmitters—a necessary process. Yet in some circumstances this process gets out of hand: Excessive enzymatic activity may abnormally deplete neurotransmitters. This is the case in some forms of clinical depression, in which the enzyme monoamine

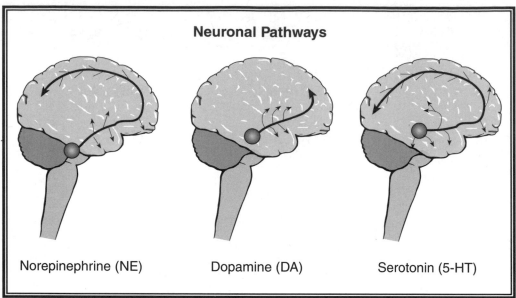

Neuronal Pathways

Norepinephrine (NE)   Dopamine (DA)   Serotonin (5-HT)

Figure 3-E

oxidase (MAO) can cause a significant inactivation of necessary neurotransmitters.

Neuroanatomy and Neurophysiology

Understanding the basic premises of neuroanatomy and neurophysiology is relevant to psychotherapists in several ways. First and foremost, an awareness of the basic principles and facts lays the groundwork for discussions of the etiologic theories of major mental illnesses. Second, this knowledge provides a foundation for understanding how psychotropic medications work. Finally, it gives the therapist the ability to answer accurately the inevitable questions that clients will pose regarding medications. Even though the responsibility for providing information about medications rests with the prescribing physician and dispensing pharmacist, therapists will nonetheless become part of the loop. Some therapists feel most comfortable referring all medication-related questions back to the physician, but others will want to assume a role of providing reassurance and feedback relevant to medication responses. In either event, solid knowledge of the facts will be of assistance.

The complexity of the entire nervous system can be overwhelming; however, having some general information is helpful. Let's begin by taking a look at the central nervous system and in particular the brain. Advances in the neurosciences, especially newer neuro-imaging techniques (such as MRI, PET, and SPECT scanning), have allowed researchers to identify more precisely which brain structures are implicated in the cognitive, perceptual, and emotional aspects of brain functioning. Likewise, such techniques have made possible the delineation of the brain structures and neurotransmitter systems that appear to malfunction in cases of primary brain pathology and in neurochemically mediated psychopathologies.

Although volumes have been written about neuroanatomy and brain functioning, in this discussion we will touch on only those brain structures felt to be relevant to the study of psychiatric disorders. What follows represents a very brief overview of functional neuroanatomy, which will lay the groundwork for the specific material presented in the chapters that follow.

Brain Structures

For practical purposes, the brain can be divided into three basic units: the brain stem and adjacent structures, the central core of the brain (including the limbic system, diencephalon, and basal ganglia), and the cerebral cortex (see figure 3-F). Clearly, the highest area of the brain, the cerebral cortex, is responsible for much of what is termed human: perception, complex cognitive processes, reality testing, initiation of behavior, judgment, and so on. Interestingly, however, the major biological dysfunctions seen in psychiatric disorders are thought to occur primarily outside of the cortex proper.

Major mental illnesses appear to involve neurochemical dysfunctions occurring in various subcortical areas: the limbic system, basal ganglia, reticular system and brain stem. These brain structures are complexly interconnected and play critical roles in mediating primary affective states and a host of biological rhythms and drives, (such as sleep, sex, hunger). Figure 3-G outlines the basic structures found in these important areas of the CNS, with reference to their various normal functions and the hypothesized psychopathology associated with each brain structure. However, it is important to note that few if any psychiatric disorders are associated with pathology or dysfunction of any single brain structure, although clearly specific neuroanatomical areas have been implicated as playing a special role in certain mental disorders.

Every region of the brain is activated and controlled by specific nerve cells. Billions of interconnecting nerve cells orchestrate the complex interactions necessary to carry out a host of functions ranging from basic instincts, reflexes, and life support, such as regulation of blood pressure, to highly developed abilities, such as abstract thought. When all works as it should, people are able to respond to physiological and psychological demands in a normal and adaptive fashion. However, brain functioning can be derailed by damage to brain tissue, via trauma, toxins, or disease, or by malfunctions occurring in nerve cells (something we will address shortly). At times such dysfunction may affect only a tiny percentage of brain neurons. (For example, in major depression the neuronal pathways affected represent only about 1 percent of total brain nerve cells. Yet the results can be devastating). The specific nature and location of brain dysfunctions will be revisited in subsequent chapters as we explore the physiological bases of major mental disorders.

Peripheral Nervous System

As figure 3-H indicates, in addition to the CNS (brain and spinal cord) the nervous system contains a further division, the peripheral nervous system (PNS). Within the PNS is the somatic division, which controls voluntary action of the skeletal muscles and carries information from sensory organs to the CNS.

A second branch of the peripheral nervous system is the autonomic nervous system (ANS). The ANS innervates involuntary organs, such as the heart, smooth muscles, and glands. Further divisions of the peripheral ANS are the sympathetic and parasympathetic systems. These systems can generally be thought of as antagonists, although this is not absolute for every activity. Most organs are innervated by both systems, and regulation is established through opposing functions.

The sympathetic nervous system (SNS) plays a role in the "fight-or-flight response." Set in motion by activity in the limbic system and hypothalamus, the sympathetic system mobilizes the body to take action in response to dangerous situations. When the fight-or-flight response is activated, there is a sudden, massive increase in metabolic rate: increased blood pressure and heart rate and the increased blood flow

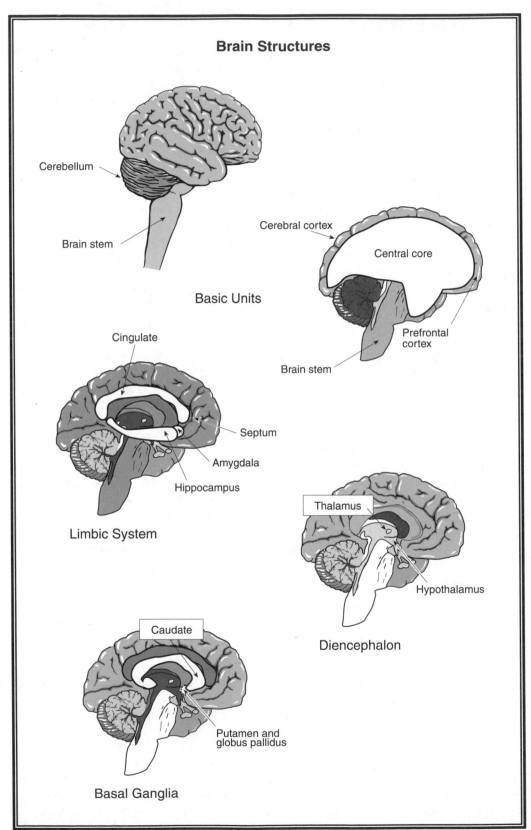

Brain Structures

Cerebellum

Brain stem

Basic Units

Cerebral cortex

Central core

Prefrontal cortex

Brain stem

Cingulate

Septum

Amygdala

Hippocampus

Limbic System

Thalamus

Hypothalamus

Diencephalon

Caudate

Putamen and globus pallidus

Basal Ganglia

Figure 3-F

Neuroanatomy, Psychological Functions, and Psychopathology

Brain Structure	Functions	Psychopathology
Cortex	Higher cognitive processing	Dementia, confusional states
Prefrontal cortex	Impulse control, attention, behavior monitoring, organization of complex information	Attention deficit disorder, schizophrenia, obsessive-compulsive disorder
Diencephalon		
thalamus	Many nerves pass through this brain structure	Not implicated in major psychiatric disorders
hypothalamus	Regulates sleep cycles, hunger, sex drive; controls endocrine and autonomic nervous system; contains pleasure centers; influences immune system	Depression, anxiety disorders
Limbic system		
amygdala	Elicits and controls aggression	Impulse control disorders, borderline personality disorder [a]
septum	Emotional and stimulus "gate," pleasure centers	Schizophrenia, impulse control disorders
cingulate	Neuronal pathways connecting limbic system structures and prefrontal lobes	Obsessive-compulsive disorder
hippocampus	Recent memory, new learning, impulse and emotional control	Alzheimer's disease, postconcussion syndrome, depression
Basal ganglia	Controls aspects of motor behavior	Parkinson's disease, antipsychotic medication side effects (extrapyramidal symptoms (EPS))
	Neuronal pathways connecting limbic system and prefrontal lobes	Obsessive-compulsive disorder
Brain stem		
reticular system	Stimulus filter or "gate"	Attention deficit disorder, schizophrenia

[a] Likely, but not proven

Figure 3-G

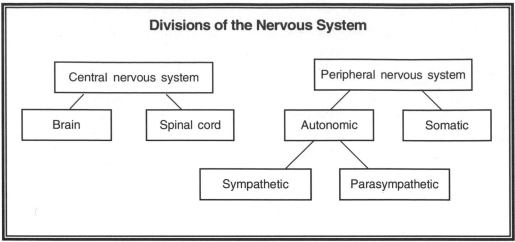

Figure 3-H

to the heart, brain, and muscles. Conversely, the parasympathetic system which is activated at times of relaxation and quiescence, acts to reduce heart rate and blood pressure in an overall attempt to conserve energy (see figure 3-I).

Many psychotropic medications can, unfortunately, affect the parasympathetic and sympathetic nervous systems—thus producing side effects. The parasympathetic system is mediated by the chemical acetylcholine. As we shall see in subsequent chapters, many psychiatric medications have anticholinergic effects (that is, they block acetylcholine) with resulting side effects (see figure 3-J). The sympathetic system is mediated primarily by norepinephrine. (Nerve cells activated by norepinephrine, epinephrine, and related compounds are called adrenergic nerves.) Certain psychotropic medications either block or activate adrenergic neurons in the SNS—again producing undesirable effects.

With this introduction completed, in part two we will begin to explore a host of clinical syndromes.

Effects of SNS and PNS Activity on Target Organs

Organ or Gland	Sympathetic Actions	Parasympathetic Actions
Pupils	Dilate	Constrict
Salivary glands	Reduce secretions	Secrete
Lungs (bronchi)	Dilate	Constrict
Heart	Increase rate	Slow rate
GI tract	Interrupt digestion	Digest
Adrenal gland	Secrete	—
Bladder	—	Empty fluids
Arteries	Constrict	Relax

Figure 3-I

Side Effects Affecting Autonomic Nervous System

Parasympathetic System—
Anticholinergic Effects

Blurry vision

Dry mouth

Constipation

Urine retention

Sympathetic System—
Adrenergic Effects

Hypotension (low norepinephrine)

Rapid heart rate (elevated
norepinephrine)

Figure 3-J

Part Two

Clinical Syndromes: Etiology, Diagnosis, and Treatment Implications

In part two of this book we address in some detail the biological etiology and differential diagnosis of major clinical syndromes. In our approach to diagnosis, we incorporate some *DSM-IV* criteria. However, at times alternative classifications and criteria are employed. Our aim is to provide a useful and clinically relevant approach that will help the therapist in decision making, particularly with regard to referral issues and medication treatments.

This section of the book begins with a chapter on preliminary diagnostic considerations. Following this are chapters addressing the most common clinical syndromes. The specifics of medication treatment (dosing, effects, side effects) will follow in part three.

4

Preliminary Diagnostic Considerations

Before launching into a detailed discussion of major psychiatric disorders, it is important to explore some preliminary diagnostic issues. These issues should be considered in the initial workup of any client for whom medications are being considered.

The most common approach to diagnosis (that of the *DSM*), and the approach we present in this book, is based on the identification of specific target symptoms that make up a particular disorder or syndrome. Such an approach certainly has merit. Yet it is crucial to keep in mind that any particular behavior, symptom, or trait *may* have diverse etiologies. That is, identical symptomatic behaviors may spring from biochemical dysfunctions, social learning experiences, or characterological sources. The three most common sources of etiologic confusion will be discussed in this chapter: the interaction between Axis I and Axis II; substance abuse and psychiatric symptomatology; and finally physical illnesses that present with cognitive, emotional, and behavioral disturbances. Successful pharmacologic treatment often depends on a thorough understanding of these important issues.

Axis I and Axis II: Complex Interactions

DSM-IV and its predecessor, *DSM-III-R*, employ a multiaxial diagnostic system. Axis I includes major psychiatric symptom disorders and syndromes, and Axis II is reserved for long-standing personality styles and disorders. This distinction between the more acute, episodic, symptomatic disorders (Axis I) and more trait-like, pervasive, and enduring personality problems (Axis II) is a useful and important advance over earlier diagnostic systems. Differentiating state and trait variables has helped researchers and clinicians alike to identify more clearly and reliably a host of psychiatric disorders. The distinction also has been useful in planning therapeutic interventions, in understanding treatment outcomes, and in making predictions about the course of disorders and their prognosis. Yet, in many respects, the boundaries between Axis I and Axis II are not entirely clear-cut. Understanding the complex interactions between Axis I and II is as important in pharmacological treatment as it is in psychotherapy. Axis I and II disorders influence one another in four common ways:

- Axis I disorder evokes Axis II characteristics

- Axis II dynamics predispose to Axis I disorders

- Axis II characteristics reflect atypical or mild chronic Axis I disorder

- Axis II dynamics influence Axis I treatment response

Let's take a look at each of these interactions.

Axis I Disorder Evokes Axis II Characteristics

Axis I disorders oftentimes enhance or exaggerate preexisting personality traits. For example, sometimes an Axis I disorder unearths behavior that was not at all evident prior to the clinical episode. The clinician may conclude that a patient has a major depression *and* a personality disorder, only to discover that the personality disorder disappears with successful treatment of the Axis I disorder. This is frequently seen in individuals diagnosed as borderline personalities in which the impact of serious depression or panic disorder results in psychological regression. During the Axis I episode there are, in fact, features verging on borderline. However, in as many as a third of such patients, with resolution of the major symptom disorder, their level of functioning resumes its normal or (more often) neurotic preclinical level. Since borderline characteristics were not evident prior to the major episode of depression or panic, and the history

---

Key Terms

Agonist. Drug or chemical that acts on a receptor to mimic the effects of a naturally occurring substance (such as a hormone or neurotransmitter), or of another chemical; for example, beta adrenergic agonist medications mimic epinephrine and produce relaxation of bronchial (lung) muscles to treat asthma.

Antagonist. Substance or drug capable of blocking (at the receptor) the activity of an agonist without exerting any effect itself. For example, antipsychotics are dopamine receptor antagonists.

Differential diagnosis. The process of considering diagnostic possibilities based on a comparison of signs and symptoms of two or more disorders or diseases.

Egodystonic. Symptoms subjectively experienced by the patient as being aversive, undesirable, or alien.

Egosyntonic. Signs or symptoms judged to be pathological by others but not experienced as distressing by the patient.

Etiology. The study of the causes of disorders and diseases.

Pathophysiology. The underlying physiological dysfunction or disease which contributes to the manifest symptoms of a disease.

continued

was not one of "stable instability," to call such a patient borderline is technically inaccurate.

Case 11

Barbara M., 35, was admitted to an inpatient psychiatric unit after she developed suicidal ideas and incidents in which she repeatedly sliced the inside of her calf. Her admitting diagnosis was major depression and borderline personality disorder. The borderline diagnosis was based on the rather bizarre self-mutilation. The treating psychiatrist informed the patient's family that her acute depression could indeed be treated, but that the apparent personality disorder would likely be a serious, ongoing problem and the prognosis was more guarded.

Barbara's history, however, failed to reveal any signs of psychiatric problems. She was a very successful owner of a small print shop and had a history of solid interpersonal relationships. Her depressive disorder occurred after her best friend had been tragically killed in a boating accident. After five days of hospitalization, she was discharged. Five weeks later, after twice weekly psychotherapy and antidepressants, she was virtually symptom-free. There was no hint of the primitive personality disturbance evident when she was first hospitalized.

> **Target symptoms.** In this book, the distinctive symptoms that are the focus (target) of medication treatment.
>
> **Toxicity.** Serious medication-related adverse effects associated with actual or potential damage to tissues, organs, or the entire body system. Toxicity may be directly related to critically elevated blood levels of a drug and may be acute (as in tricyclic antidepressant overdose) or chronic (as in prolonged, moderately elevated lithium level). A drug may also produce "toxic effects" at therapeutic doses (such as phenothiazine's potential for inducing bone marrow damage, which in turn causes decreased production of white blood cells).

Another common example is when a very severe depression or anxiety disorder pulls the rug out from under a person. As a result, we may see the emergence of helplessness and overly dependent behavior. This *may* be an exaggeration of preexisting dependent traits, but it may also be the kind of regressive behavior seen across many personality styles when one is laid low by a serious, debilitating illness.

Axis II Dynamics Predispose to Axis I Disorders

Certain personality disorders may predispose an individual to increased risk of developing an Axis I disorder. We can see this emerge in at least two ways. First, people with personality disorders often, if not always, experience particular, unique areas of emotional vulnerability. For example, histrionic, dependent, avoidant, and many borderline patients have strong dependency longings and an exquisite sensitivity to separation stresses. As a group, these people are at higher risk for developing major depressions, serious anxiety reactions, or both in the wake of interpersonal losses. For these patients, relatively minor social rebuffs, rejections, or losses may precipitate significant depressive reactions. In a parallel manner, obsessive and paranoid personalities highly value being in control. Even minor life stresses that decrease one's sense of control or predictability can plunge these people into states of high anxiety, hypervigilance, and ruminative self doubt.

A second way Axis II problems can increase risk is that repetitive maladaptive behavior patterns can result in recurring interpersonal stressors. For example, the clinging, overly dependent personality may, by his or her interpersonal style, repeatedly drive people away. Here the maladaptive behavior provokes numerous rejections, which in turn can lead to episodes of depression.

Thus, when medications are used to treat various Axis I disorders, it is well to keep in mind that, despite the success of drug treatment, ultimate therapeutic success and relapse prevention may depend heavily on the role Axis II factors play.

Axis II Characteristics Reflect Axis I Disorder

It is possible that what initially appear to be characteristic symptoms of personality disorder may reflect some form of mild, chronic, or atypical Axis I disorder. Let's consider several examples. For years clinicians described certain patients as suffering from masochistic or depressive personalities. These people were often seen as chronically pessimistic, bitter, irritable individuals, and the implication was that the low-grade depressive traits were manifestations of personality—that is, etched into the character of the individual. Although certainly this is the case for some people, in recent years a significant number of dysthymic patients have experienced very positive results when treated with antidepressants.

These so-called depressive characters likely have suffered from a form of chronic, low-grade biological depression. Similarly, recent reports of successful treatment of social anxiety in "avoidant personalities" using MAO inhibitors may indicate another group of patients whose character pathology seems to be rooted in a type of biochemical disturbance.

Undoubtedly, many people presenting with personality problems are best understood as exhibiting true disorders of character, and for these people medication treatment is not appropriate. However, it is very important not to conclude automatically that such behaviors are solely attributable to character pathology (see figure 4-A). Certain behavioral characteristics or traits seen in various personality disorders *may* be due to subtle neurochemical malfunction, which may respond to medication.

Just because a trait is long-standing, it is not appropriate to automatically assume that it is truly characterological. Figure 4-A can serve as a reminder to consider the *possibility* that certain characteristics may be due to chronic biochemical dysfunction. (See interesting discussions of this topic in Peter Kramer's best-selling book, *Listening to Prozac* 1993.)

Axis II Dynamics Influence Axis I Treatment Response

As mentioned in chapter 2, individuals' particular personality style and unique psychodynamics will often dramatically influence how they respond to pharmacotherapy. Robert Michaels (1992) has recently commented that in general clinical practice two-thirds of patients with Axis I disorders appear to respond quite well either to medication treatment or to brief, targeted psychological interventions, such as cognitive-behavioral or interpersonal therapy. However, a significant minority of patients with clear-cut Axis I disorders don't respond well to such treatments, primarily due to serious co-morbid character pathology. In treating these people, at the very least the clinician must be alert to how personality factors influence treatment outcome; often medication treatment must be accompanied by more intensive psychotherapy that addresses the personality disorder.

Personality Traits That May Reflect Biochemical Disorders

Axis II Traits	Medication-Responsive Axis I Disorder	Psychotropic Medication Options
Chronic boredom; emptiness; irritability; hypochrodriasis; low energy; chronic fatigue; pessimism, negative thinking; feelings of shame, humiliation	Depression	Antidepressants
Easily hurt by criticism; helplessness, dependency; difficulty making decisions	Depression, anxiety disorders	Antidepressants
Social anxiety, avoidance	Social phobia, panic disorder	Antidepressants, beta blockers, benzodiazepines
Magical thinking; odd speech	Psychotic disorders	Antipsychotics
Excessive worry	Generalized anxiety disorders	Antidepressants, buspirone, benzodiazepines
Impulsiveness; stimulus seeking; affective instability	Attention deficit disorder, bipolar disorder	Stimulants, antidepressants, lithium
Separation stress; nonassertivenes	Anxiety disorders	Antidepressants, benzodiazepines
Perfectionism; preoccupation with rules, order, details, lists or cleanliness; workaholic	Obsessive-compulsive disorder	Antidepressants (5-HT type)

Figure 4-A

Substance Abuse

Substance abuse can directly cause or contribute to a wide array of psychiatric symptoms: depression, anxiety disorders, psychosis, mania, and so on. Not only can the use of recreational drugs produce psychological symptoms, but frequently such substances markedly interfere with psychological or psychiatric treatment. A common example of this occurs when moderate-to-heavy alcohol use adversely affects liver functioning, causing prescribed psychotropic medications to be inadequately metabolized. The result can be inadequate blood levels of the medication, as in the following case.

Case 12

Jerry H. was first seen for psychiatric consultation six months ago. He presented with a classic major depression, which had emerged during an especially difficult marital separation and divorce. Jerry had initially reported only occasional social drinking, "a few times a month." After five months of psychotherapy and aggressive antidepressant treatment he was still quite depressed. Three antidepressant medications had been tried in conjunction with cognitive-behavioral psychotherapy, with little improvement. It was eventually learned that Jerry actually had been consuming four to six beers every night. Three weeks after the alcohol use had been curtailed he began to show his first positive response to the antidepressant. The alcohol use (unknown to the therapist for five months) had been the main culprit in preventing antidepressants from ever reaching adequate blood levels.

Although a very wide range of prescription and nonprescription drugs can cause psychiatric symptoms, the two most commonly encountered in clinical practice are alcohol and caffeine. (In subsequent clinical chapters additional specific drugs will be listed as they contribute to particular psychiatric disorders.) It is always important to get a complete drug history on each person being evaluated.

In general, more than 1.5 ounces of alcohol (or the equivalent: one beer, or one glass of wine) per day, may directly contribute to psychiatric symptoms, may interfere with proper metabolism of psychotropic medications, or both. Obviously, excessive use often leads to two additional complications: addiction or dependence and the use of the drug as a means of acting out (emotional numbing), which can interfere with the process of self-exploration, abreaction, or "working through" in psychotherapy. Appropriate psychotherapy and pharmacotherapy can (and often do) fail because of ongoing and often unrecognized substance abuse.

In general, over 250 mg (especially amounts over 500 mg) of caffeine per day can cause or contribute to psychiatric symptoms, especially anxiety, irritability, sleep disturbance, and agitation. Figure 4-B provides a guideline for a caffeine history—which should be done on every person being evaluated.

Physical Illness

A number of investigators have found that a rather substantial minority of people seeking psychiatric services are actually suffering from undiagnosed physical illness. The primary medical disorder either causes or contributes to the emergence of psychiatric symptoms. Let's sample a couple of studies: Hall et al. (1978) carefully evaluated 658 consecutive psychiatric outpatients. These researchers found that 9 percent had medical disorders that were the primary cause of psychiatric symptoms. Koran

Caffeine Content of Common Substances

Beverages			Over-the-Counter Drugs	
Coffee,	6 oz	150 mg	Appetite-control pills	100–200 mg
Decaf coffee	6 oz	5 mg	NoDoz	100 mg
Tea	6 oz	50 mg	Vivarin	200 mg
Hot cocoa	6 oz	15 mg	Anacin	32 mg
Soft drinks	12 oz	40–60 mg	Excedrin	65 mg
(colas, Mountain			Midol	132 mg
Dew, Mr. Pibb,			Vanquish	33 mg
Mello Yello, Dr.			Triaminicin	30 mg
Pepper, Big Red)			Dristan	16 mg

Prescription Drugs

Cafergot	100 mg
Fiorinal	140 mg
Darvon compound	32 mg

Source: FDA National Center: Drugs and Biologics (as cited in Avis 1993).

Figure 4-B

et al. (1989) found an even higher number of psychiatric patients with underlying medical disorders—17 percent.

Robert Taylor (1990) has aptly referred to such cases as "psychological masquerade." Here, unrecognized medical disorders either directly or indirectly affect the biochemistry of the brain and produce a host of emotional, cognitive, and behavioral symptoms.

It is crucial to identify those people suffering from psychological masquerade for two reasons: Firstly, various medical illnesses need to be treated early. Failure to recognize and treat them may result in prolonged suffering, permanent impairment, progressive physical decline, and, at times, death. Second, one's best efforts at providing psychological treatment may be in vain if the underlying medical condition goes unrecognized. However, nonmedical therapists are not trained in medical diagnosis. So what steps can they take to identify those patients who have a physical illness?

The role of the nonmedical therapist is not to make definitive medical diagnoses, but rather to be alert to certain warning signs that may signal the presence of a physical illness or that at least increase one's index of suspicion. Obviously, when a medical illness is suspected, a referral to a physician or emergency medical facility is in order.

For practical purposes we can divide medical illnesses with psychiatric symptomatology into three categories:

- Illnesses and conditions that do not directly affect the CNS, but can lead to secondary (reactive) emotional responses. These conditions are generally recognized and reported by the patient. Examples are a person who develops a serious reactive depression after sustaining a spinal cord injury and paralysis and an individual who is diagnosed with glaucoma and may be facing blindness.

- Illnesses and conditions that affect the CNS and impair cognitive functioning. These conditions are of greatest importance—where the medical problem may go unnoticed and what predominates are psychiatric symptoms.

- Illnesses and conditions that affect neurochemistry, but do not affect cognitive functioning. The latter two conditions include primary disorders of the nervous system (such as brain tumors and degenerative diseases) and a host of systemic illnesses that indirectly influence brain chemistry.

Illnesses and Conditions Affecting Cognitive Functioning

Disorders affecting cognitive functioning can be further subdivided into: acute and chronic or insidious categories. Acute disorders tend to have a more profound effect on brain functioning and have an impact on the following cognitive functions:

- Patients may appear to be drowsy and suffer from what is called "clouding of consciousness."

- Attention and concentration may be impaired.

- Speech may be slurred.

- Content of speech may reveal confused and disorganized thinking.

- Gait may be unsteady.

- The person can become disoriented.

- Recent memory (the ability for new learning and recall) is impaired.

- There may be agitation and/or labile emotions.

These areas of functioning can be evaluated by the use of a brief neuro-cognitive mental status exam (see appendix E). Acute disorders affecting the CNS have mul-

---

Acute Organic Brain Syndromes

- Anoxia
- CNS infections
- CVA (strokes), hemorrhages
- Head injuries
- Metabolic disorders such as hypoglycemia, adrenal disease, vitamin deficiencies, electrolyte imbalances
- Organ diseases such as hepatic encephalopathy
- Pernicious anemia
- Toxic reactions, such as drug interactions or overdoses

Figure 4-C

Causes of Chronic Organic Brain Syndromes

- AIDS or HIV dementia
- Alzheimer's disease
- Chronic sequelae of head injury
- Cognitive disorders associated with chronic substance abuse
- Huntington's chorea

- Multi-infarct disorder
- Multiple sclerosis
- Neoplasms (CNS tumors)
- Parkinson's disease
- Pick's disease
- Wilson's disease

Figure 4-D

tiple etiologies (see figure 4-C). Many of these conditions can be potentially life threatening, thus immediate medical attention is indicated.

Chronic, insidious brain syndromes usually do not present with a clouding of consciousness; patients appear fully awake. Also, disturbances in gait and slurred speech are *generally* not seen. (Exceptions do exist, however. For instance, in Parkinson's disease there is a gait disturbance.) The onset of symptoms is gradual. Hallmark symptoms usually include: impaired recent memory, poor ability to reproduce geometric designs, impaired concentration, and an erosion of higher level cognitive abilities (such as impaired reasoning and judgment). These disorders can also be evaluated using the brief neuro-cognitive mental status exam in appendix E, and by taking a complete history from the patient and an informed relative. If a chronic brain syndrome is suspected, a medical referral is indicated. Figure 4-D lists causes of common chronic brain syndromes.

Illnesses and Conditions Affecting Neurochemistry

There are a number of medical disorders that have little or no effect on cognitive function but can adversely affect the biochemistry of the limbic system and other subcortical brain areas. Thus, although individuals suffering from these conditions may appear intact on the brief neuro-cognitive mental status exam, they may exhibit

---

Medical Illness Checklist

- Onset of psychiatric symptoms has "come out of the blue"—not precipitated by identifiable psychosocial stressors.

- The patient is over 55, thus at increased risk for a host of medical illnesses.

- The patient takes multiple medications—which may interact adversely.

- No personal or family history of similar psychiatric symptoms.

- Recent history of head injury.

- Hallucinations or illusions—especially visual, olfactory, tactile, or gustatory (such perceptual disturbances are indicative of neurologic disease).

- The patient looks physically ill or has abnormal vital signs (such as very low blood pressure, fever, weak pulse).

Source: Taylor 1990

Figure 4-E

Specific Physical Symptoms Checklist

Physical Symptoms	Psychiatric Symptoms	Possible Disorder
Abdominal pain, jaundice, constipation	Depression	Pancreatic cancer
Weight gain, cold intolerance, dry skin, hair loss, puffy face, fatigue	Depression, psychosis	Hypothyroidism
Weight loss, heat intolerance, sweating, tremors, wide-eyed state	Anxiety, agitated depression	Hyperthyroidism
Bad breath, urine odor, frequent urination	Depression	Diabetes mellitus
Weakness, dizziness, lightheadedness, sweating, tremors	Anxiety (acute onset)	Hypoglycemia
Muscular weakness, fatigue	Depression	Myasthenia gravis
Sensory disturbances, paresthesia, transient motor disturbances	Depression, euphoria, conversion symptoms	Multiple sclerosis
Weakness, fatigue, diffuse pain, incoordination	Depression, impaired memory	Pernicious anemia
Abdominal pain, weakness, confusion after ingestion of alcohol or barbituates	Anxiety	Porphyria
Increased skin pigmentation, weight loss, diarrhea, muscle cramps, low blood pressure	Depression	Hypoadrenalism (Addison's disease)
Muscle weakness, moon face, hirsutism, hypertension	Irritability, euphoria, depression	Hyperadrenalism (Cushing's disease)
Hypertension, headache	Anxiety	Pheochromocytoma (adrenal gland tumor)
Fever, malaise	Depression, agitation	Viral or bacterial infection
Fatigue, joint pain	Depression	Various rheumatoid disorders (e.g. fibromyalgia), chronic fatigue syndromes
Headaches, weakness	Depression, mania, personality changes	Brain tumor
Any physical symptoms	Any psychiatric disorder	Drug effects or side effects

Note: This listing does not cover all possible medical disorders that may cause psychiatric symptoms; however, these do represent those most commonly encountered in clinical practice.

Figure 4-F

pronounced psychiatric symptoms as the systemic medical illness dysregulates the chemistry of the brain.

How might the nonmedical therapist detect the presence of such medical disorder? We will look at two approaches: to evaluate for global warning signs (see figure 4-E), and to ask about particular physical symptoms (see figure 4-F). In each case, the clinician should do a brief overview of various signs and physical symptoms. The goal again is not to make a medical diagnosis but rather to either raise or lower one's index of suspicion. If a medical condition is suspected, a referral for appropriate medical care is indicated.

Many of the symptoms listed in figure 4-F are fairly nonspecific and may be elicited from many patients, but some particular physical symptoms should raise your index of suspicion, such as when there are several physical complaints, not just a simple nonspecific complaint like fatigue. When in doubt, refer for evaluation. In fact, it is probably advisable that anyone with a significant psychiatric disorder have a medical evaluation.

Keep in mind that medications and other drugs are a very common cause of emotional symptoms—this includes prescription, nonprescription, and other recreational drugs and alcohol. Obtaining collateral history from family members may be helpful. Also conducting the "bag test"—having the person bring in *all* (this cannot be stressed too much) medications he or she is taking for the therapist to see and make a record of.

In summary, after assessing for the presence of Axis II characteristics and understanding how these may influence the primary symptom disorders, and after ruling in or out substance abuse and coexisting medical illnesses, the clinician is ready to formulate a clinical diagnosis. The following chapters address major diagnostic groups with a focus on clinical presentation, differential diagnosis, etiology, and treatment decision making. In each area we pay particular attention to which diagnostic characteristics indicate the need for psychotropic medication treatment.

5

Depressive Disorders

Depressive disorders (also often referred to as affective or mood disorders) represent an extremely broad, heterogeneous group of disorders. These clinical syndromes share some common symptoms (especially dysphoria), but in fact reflect a number of disorders that have diverse etiologies: characterological, acute reactive, and biologic. (Note that bipolar disorder, or manic-depressive illness, is covered separately, in chapter 6.) The symptoms, course, prognosis, and response to treatment vary considerably depending on the particular type of depressive disorder seen clinically; thus a solid understanding of the differential diagnosis is crucial for treatment-oriented decision making.

Differential Diagnosis

It is helpful to first view depressive disorders as falling broadly into three primary groups: reactive sadness, grief, and clinical depression.

Reactive sadness is characterized by relatively low-grade mood changes—sadness, disappointment, despair—that occur in response to minor losses and disappointments. The emotional responses are considered to be normal and appropriate. They are transient, and, most importantly, these mood disturbances do not typically interfere with functioning; that is, they have little impact on academic, occupational, or social or interpersonal functioning.

Grief, or uncomplicated bereavement, can be a much more prolonged and intensely painful experience. Grief is a normal and emotionally necessary response to major losses, such as death of a loved one or divorce. Most normal grief reactions result in significant degrees of emotional distress for a period of six to twelve months and continued, albeit less intense, grieving often lasts for an additional one to three years. Social and occupational functioning can be derailed for a while, although most people experiencing a grief reaction do continue to work and socialize.

There are two important features that distinguish grief from clinical depression. First, as noted in Freud's classic, "Mourning and Melancholia" (1917), with grief, self-esteem remains relatively intact, despite significant dysphoria. Second, as painful as it is, the grieving process is healthy and adaptive; it is an active process of mourning that eventually leads to emotional healing. In clinical depressions self-esteem almost always erodes, and true depression is a clearly pathological condition.

Certainly, what appears initially to be a grief reaction often disintegrates into a true clinical depression, so the boundary between these disorders is not always sharply defined. When the following symptoms emerge in the wake of a serious loss, this signals that normal grief has evolved into a clinical depression:

When Grief Becomes Clinical Depression

- Marked erosion of self-esteem
- Agitation*
- Early morning awakening*
- Serious weight loss*
- Suicidal ideation or attempts
- Anhedonia (loss of the ability to experience any pleasure)*
- Marked impairment of social, interpersonal, academic, or occupational functioning

* When this clinical picture emerges, psychotherapy, psychotropic medication treatment, or both, become necessary. These symptoms marked with an asterisk are targets for antidepressant medications.

The vast majority of individuals encountering uncomplicated bereavement do not need psychological or psychiatric treatment. However, it is estimated that about 15 percent of individuals do in fact develop a clinical depression following a major loss.

Clinical depressions are characterized by their intensity, duration, impact on functioning, and a host of symptoms. Most true clinical depressions result in tremendous personal suffering, can last for months to years (left untreated), and normal daily functioning is severely affected.

We can further divide *clinical depressions* into the following categories:

Types of Clinical Depression

- *Major unipolar depressions:* reactive, biological, reactive-biological, atypical
- *Bipolar disorder:* manic and depressive episodes (see chapter 6)
- *"Minor" depressions:* dysthymia, chronic residuals of partially recovered major depressions

---

Major Unipolar Depressions

For practical purposes and to aid in treatment decision making, it is useful to conceptualize three primary types and one atypical version of major depression. All have in common marked impairment in functioning, a typically long duration, and one or all of the core symptoms listed below:

Core Symptoms Common to All Depressions

- Mood of sadness, despair, emptiness
- Anhedonia (loss of the ability to experience pleasure)
- Low self-esteem
- Apathy, low motivation, and social withdrawal
- Excessive emotional sensitivity
- Negative, pessimistic thinking
- Irritability
- Suicidal ideas

Note: Some degree of decreased capacity for pleasure (anhedonia) may be seen in all types of depression. In depressions that involve a biochemical disturbance, this loss of ability to experience pleasure can become so pronounced that the patient has almost no moments of joy or pleasure. Such people are said to have a "nonreactive mood," which means that they are unable to get out of their depressed mood even temporarily.

Reactive depressions

Classic reactive depressions (sometimes referred to as psychological depressions) can range in intensity from mild or moderate (for example, adjustment disorders with depressed mood) to severe (major depression). These disorders occur in response to identifiable psychosocial stressors. These stressors may be acute and intense (such as loss of a loved one), insidious (as in the case of a gradual deterioration in the quality of marital relationship), or in the distant past (for example, the emotions experienced by a survivor of child abuse who in adulthood begins to recall long-forgotten abusive events).

In its pure form, reactive depression can present with severe levels of symptomatology, yet basic physical functions (sleep, energy levels, and so on) are relatively unaffected. Note that many reactive depressions do take on biological features, as will be described below, but the pure reactive disorder noted here is seen without major physiological symptoms.

Depression Facts

- Lifetime prevalence for depressive disorders is 19 percent.

- Suicide rate for patients with major depression is 15 percent.

- 17 million people per year suffer from major depression in the United States. Another 7.5 million experience chronic low-grade depression.

- The incidence of depression ratio of women to men is 2:1.

- Only one in three Americans who suffers a bout of major depression seeks treatment. Yet treatment is effective in up to 80 percent of depressed patients—even those suffering with very severe depressions.

Medical Disorders That Can Cause Depression

- Addison's disease
- AIDS
- Anemia
- Asthma
- Chronic fatigue syndrome
- Chronic infection (mononucleosis, tuberculosis)
- Chronic pain
- Congestive heart failure
- Cushing's disease
- Diabetes
- Hypothyroidism
- Infectious hepatitis
- Influenza
- Malignancies (cancer)
- Malnutrition
- Multiple sclerosis
- Porphyria
- Rheumatoid arthritis
- Syphilis
- Systemic lupus erythematosus
- Ulcerative colitis
- Uremia

Figure 5-A

Drugs That Can Cause Depression

Type	Generic name	Brand name
Alcohol	Wine, beer, spirits	Various brands
Antianxiety drugs	Diazepam	Valium
	Chlordiazepoxide	Librium
Antihypertensives (for high blood pressure)	Reserpine	Serpasil, Ser-Ap-Es
	Propranolol hydrochloride	Inderal
	Methyldopa	Aldomet
	Guanethidine sulfate	Ismelin sulfate
	Clonidine hydrochloride	Catapres
	Hydralazine hydrochloride	Apresoline hydrochloride
Antiparkinsonian drugs	Levodopa carbidopa	Sinemet
	Levodopa	
	Amantadine hydrochloride	Dupar, Larodopa Symmetrel
Birth control pills	Progestin-estrogen combination	Various brands
Corticosteroids and other hormones	Cortisone acetate	Cortone
	Estrogen	Premarin, Ogen, Estrace, Estraderm
	Progesterone and derivatives	Provera, Depo-Provera, Norlutate, Norplant, Progestasert

Figure 5-B

Biological depressions

Biologically based depressive disorders, in their purest form, are not seen as a reaction to stressors. In fact, they can emerge apparently spontaneously, "out of the blue"—in individuals encountering little in terms of life stress. The trigger for biological depressions can be traced to any of a number of conditions that alter neurotransmitter function in key areas of the limbic system. The conditions responsible for biological depressions fall into four categories:

- Medical illnesses that lead to systemic changes and ultimately to brain dysfunction (see figure 5-A).

- Female sex-hormone fluctuation, especially noted postpartum, during menopause, and premenstrually.

- Medications and recreational drugs (see Figure 5-B). (Note that alcohol and minor tranquilizers are often used or abused during times of emotional stress, and, almost invariably, eventually make depression worse.)

- Endogenous biological depressions. These disorders appear to emerge spontaneously in certain at-risk individuals, in the absence of stressful events. The prevailing theory (discussed below) is that such disorders likely reflect a genetically transmitted biologic vulnerability that leads to repeated dysfunction of selected neurons in the limbic system and resulting recurring depressive episodes.

In experimental settings, researchers have been able to identify some biological markers for these disorders, including reduced frontal cortex metabolic activity, abnormalities shown on sleep EEGs, and neurotransmitter metabolite irregularities in cerebral spinal fluid. However, for practical, economic, and safety reasons, such tests are not used in clinical settings. What have been and continue to be the most reliable markers of biological depression are the emergence of depression in the absence of identifiable psychosocial stressors *and* the presence of any of the following physiological symptoms:

Physiological Symptoms of Depression

- Appetite disturbance—decreased or increased, with accompanying weight loss or gain.

- Fatigue.

- Decreased sex drive.

- Restlessness, agitation, or psychomotor retardation.

- Diurnal variations in mood—usually feeling worse in the morning.

- Impaired concentration and forgetfulness.

- Pronounced anhedonia—total loss of the ability to experience pleasure.

- Sleep disturbance—early morning awakening, frequent awakenings throughout the night; occasionally hypersomnia (excessive sleeping). Note that initial insomnia (difficulty in falling asleep) may be seen with depression, but is not diagnostic of a major depressive disorder. Initial insomnia can be seen anyone experiencing stress in general. Initial insomnia alone is more characteristic of anxiety disorders than of depression.

These symptoms are commonly referred to as *vegetative* or *neurovegetative* symptoms. Not only are these symptoms a marker of biological depression, they also serve as our major target symptoms—alerting the therapist that the patient should be referred for antidepressant medication treatment.

Typically, for the diagnosis to be more definitive, the patient must have one or more of these symptoms on a sustained basis: present most days for a period of at least two weeks. Sporadic or occasional vegetative symptoms may hint at a neurotransmitter abnormality, but do not suggest an entrenched clinical depression.

Reactive-biological depression

Sometimes referred to as endogenomorphic depressions, reactive-biological depressions represent a very large number of the depressions seen clinically. These disorders begin in much the same way as the more classic reactive depressions described above. However, with time, we see the emergence of various physiological symptoms. These disorders are not truly endogenous; however, at some point the effects of psychological stress appear to adversely influence brain functioning. What emerges is a sort of mixed depression—with both psychological-reactive and biologic symptoms.

Atypical depressions

Atypical depression, or hysteroid-dysphoria as it is sometimes called, is a subtype of major depression characterized by the following symptoms:

Symptoms of Atypical Depression

- Reactive dysphoria—sadness or despair comes and goes in response to psychological stressors

- Profound fatigue, low energy

- Hypersomnia (excessive sleeping)

- Increased appetite and weight gain

- Sensitivity to interpersonal rejection or separation

- Phobias and panic attacks

As we will see later, this type of depressive disorder has been shown to be effectively treated with a particular subtype of antidepressants called monoamine oxidase inhibitors (MAOIs). Recent findings suggest that atypical depressions may also respond to selective serotonin re-uptake inhibitors (SSRIs).

Efficacy of medication treatment

Major depressions can certainly occur once and never again. Yet, 66 percent of people experiencing a major depression encounter recurring episodes (on average, six per lifetime). Thus treatment and resolution of the current episode is crucial, but relapse prevention is also an important treatment goal. The eventual suicide rate for individuals with major depression is 15 percent. The economic burden to society is staggering: Direct and indirect costs are estimated to be $16 billion per year in the United States (Stoudemire et al. 1986), not to mention the incalculable personal suffering of patients and their families. Good patient education especially focused on the early signs of recurrence can go far to avert future episodes.

There is a large body of research supporting the finding that, when physiological symptoms are present, antidepressant medications are quite effective. Presumably the presentation of the symptoms listed above (physiological and atypical) signals the presence of an underlying dysregulation of particular neurotransmitters, especially norepinephrine, serotonin, or both. These symptoms continue to be our most reliable behavioral markers of an underlying biological dysfunction. Thus very few people suffering from pure reactive-psychological depressions benefit from antidepressant medication treatment. However, improvement rates for the more physiologically based disorders (biological, reactive-biological, and atypical depressions) when treated with antidepressants are as high as 80 percent.[1] Thus, the presence of the sustained physiological symptoms listed above can serve as primary target symptoms for antidepressant medication treatment.

It is very important to note that medical treatment of depression focuses primarily on restoring normal biological functioning (that is, improvement in physiological symptoms) and only secondarily affects mood, self esteem, and so forth.

Psychotic Depressions

Major depression and bipolar illness (the subject of chapter 6) can, if extremely severe, manifest psychotic symptoms. Typically, the hallucinations and delusions seen in psychotic mood disorders are said to be "mood congruent," which means that the themes of these symptoms are congruent with the dominant mood. For example, a psychotically depressed patient might have delusions that she is the most disgusting or evil person in the world and should be executed. This delusional belief embodies the depressive themes of extremely low self-esteem and guilt. Compare this to schizophrenic symptoms, which most often are bizarre and unconnected to a dominant mood state, for example, the anxious man who believes a radio transmitter has been implanted in his thumb so that neighbors can hear broadcasts of his inner thoughts.

When symptoms of major depression and psychosis coexist, medication treatment is always warranted. (Often hospitalization, ECT, or both may also be necessary.) Psychotically depressed patients do not respond to psychotherapy alone, and they represent a *very* high suicide risk when actively psychotic. It has been firmly documented that treatment with antidepressants alone is not very effective (only 25 percent). Likewise, treatment with antipsychotics alone produce disappointing results (35 percent effective). However, combined antidepressant-antipsychotic treatment is significantly more effective (60 to 70 percent). Electroconvulsive treatment is really the gold standard in the treatment of psychotic mood disorders (90 percent effective). (See chapters 14 and 17, on treatment with antidepressants and antipsychotics, respectively.)

---

1. The high improvement rates are seen in those individuals for whom the diagnosis is correct and for whom treatment is appropriately managed. Diagnostic and treatment errors abound, and in general clinical practice success rates usually fall below 80 percent.

"Minor" Depressions

The depressive disorders described below are sometimes referred to as minor depressions because they do not reach the depths or intensity seen in major depression. However, the term *minor* may be a misnomer. Although these disorders are low-grade, they tend to be very long-term, often having their onset in late childhood or early adolescence, and potentially lasting a lifetime. The cumulative toll such disorders exact on the quality of life and productivity over a lifetime are not minor at all! These chronic, low-grade depressions fall into two categories: dysthymia and chronic residuals of partially recovered major depression.

Dysthymia is characterized by the following symptoms:

Dysthymic Symptoms

Core Psychological Symptoms

Low-grade sadness
Irritability
Negative thinking
Low self-esteem

Possible Biologic Symptoms

Low energy
Decreased capacity to experience
    pleasure

Note: These biologic symptoms may be considered as targets for medication treatment.

Unfortunately dysthymic individuals can also suffer not only from chronic, low-grade depression but also from periods of major depression. These more severe episodes are superimposed on the chronic depression, and often, upon recovery from the major episode, the patient returns to his or her preclinical norm: low-grade depression. Such disorders have been termed "double depression" (see figure 5-C).

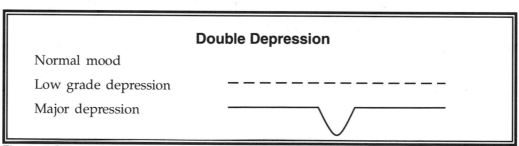

Figure 5-C

These minor depressions have long been seen as characterological and difficult to treat. However, during the past decade a large number of studies conclude that 50 to 55 percent of dysthymic patients do respond, and respond well, to treatment with antidepressants. (For review articles see Stewart, Quitkin, and Klein 1992 and Akiskal and Weise 1992.) It is likely, based on these findings, that approximately one-half of dysthymic patients may, in fact, be suffering from a type of chronic low-grade biologic depression. The other half may be experiencing more of a true characterological depression. For example, in unpublished data, Nicholas Ward (1992) finds that a history of serious early child abuse (emotional, sexual, or physical) in the context of dysthymia does not portend well for a good response to antidepressants (only about 15 percent respond). This finding should *not* preclude the use of antidepressants in survivors of child abuse, but rather serves to highlight the possibility that this version of dysthymia may issue more from pervasively tragic life circumstances than from disordered neurotransmitters.

A final type of minor depression is seen in those 15 to 20 percent of individuals who experience only a partial remission of symptoms following a major depressive episode. These people may clinically *look* dysthymic but are not. Typically, they do not have a lifelong history of low-grade or characterological depression. Usually these patients need ongoing and often more aggressive treatment to truly resolve the persistent depressive symptoms.

Etiology

It is easy to be seduced by surface symptoms and make assumptions about etiology and treatment. If all sore throats were treated with antibiotics, only about 15 to 20 percent would respond because most sore throats are due to viral rather than bacterial infections. Likewise with psychiatric disorders: Common symptoms should not automatically lead to conclusions regarding common etiologies.

The causes of depression have been viewed from a number of developmental and psychological perspectives, including the following:

- Psychodynamic models focusing on retroflexed rage and inadequate psychological "metabolism" of aggression and the development of an overly punitive superego

- Attachment theories and the role that loss plays in precipitating depression or mourning, in humans and in animals (Bowlby)

- Object relations theory, which implicates faulty separation-individuation experiences and a failure to develop self-soothing introjects (Mahler and others)

- The learned helplessness model, in which depression is seen to emerge when people (or animals) perceive that "No matter what I do, I have no ability to influence aversive experiences" (Seligman)

- The cognitive model, in which certain life experiences contribute to the development of pervasive cognitive schemas or cognitive distortions—negative mental sets and expectations that automatically influence ongoing perceptions, conclusions, and predictions about the future (Beck, Ellis)

Clearly, these models all have merit in helping to tease out complex factors that can contribute to the development of depression. These psychological causes also very likely influence much of what goes on in the so-called biologic depressions. However, the focus of this section is limited to a discussion of current theories of biological causation—causes that either underlie or contribute to the development of the biologic-based depressions listed above.

The dominant theories of biologic causation draw from a diverse source of research, which will be highlighted only briefly here:

- Genetic studies (primarily derived from population, family, twin, and adoptive studies) suggest that certain depressive disorders may have a genetic loading, especially bipolar and unipolar depression.

- PET scan studies revealing brain metabolic rates have indicated decreased levels of glucose metabolism in the lateral prefrontal cortex in patients with major depression (Baxter 1991).

- Assays of neurotransmitter derivatives (metabolites: HIAA from serotonin and MHPG from norepinephrine) in blood, urine, and cerebral spinal fluid have found abnormally low levels of these important neurotransmitters during major depressive episodes.

- Sleep-EEG studies have documented abnormal sleep patterns in depressed patients, especially a tendency to rapidly enter the first stage of REM early in the sleep cycle.

- Many depressed patients show evidence of abnormal hormone levels, especially adrenocortical hormones, which are adversely influenced by neurotransmitter dysfunction in the limbic system and hypothalamus.

Monoamine Hypothesis

This data, coupled with numerous positive outcome studies of the effectiveness of antidepressants, has led to the development of the *monoamine* (or biogenic amine) *hypothesis* of depression. The theory holds that depressive symptoms are ushered in by a malfunction of either norepinephrine (NE) or serotonin (5-HT) neurons, which play critical roles in the functioning of the limbic system and the adjacent hypothalamus. The basic neuronal malfunction is felt to be identical for either NE or 5-HT neurons, thus what follows (a description of the pathophysiology of NE neurons) can also be seen to occur in individuals in whom 5-HT neurons are affected. For reasons that are not well understood, patients with major depression (with vegetative symptoms) appear to suffer from either NE or 5-HT dysfunction, but probably not both simultaneously (although some exceptions exist).

Recall the discussion in chapter 3 of normal chemical events at the level of the synapse. The monoamine hypothesis holds that two abnormalities develop in NE or 5-HT neurons in the brain. The first is excessive re-uptake (see figure 5-D). The effect of this abnormality is that significant amounts of neurotransmitter—already released from the presynaptic cell—are rapidly reabsorbed. The result is decreased ability to stimulate postsynaptic excitatory receptors. The nerve cells, in a sense, are unplugged. A second condition arises with time: the up-regulating (increased production) of *inhibitory* receptors. The result is decreased cellular excitability. These two processes operate together to reduce neuronal firing dramatically.

This condition comes to affect thousands of NE or 5-HT cells throughout the limbic system and hypothalamus. Biologic rhythms (such as sleep cycles) and drives including hunger and sex drive, get off track; pleasure centers fail to respond (anhedonia); and emotional-control structures in the limbic system fail (resulting in lability or emotional dyscontrol). With time the emergence of neurovegetative symptoms is seen. Without treatment, this abnormal condition can persist for many months (on average six to eighteen months), and then it begins to reestablish normal functioning—that is, the condition is often self-limiting—again for reasons that are not well understood.

Another way *both* NE and 5-HT cells can shut down is when the naturally occurring enzyme, monoamine oxidase (MAO) becomes too active, excessively degrading neurotransmitters. This results in major depression, but often a depression with its own unique symptomatic signature (see "Atypical depression," above).

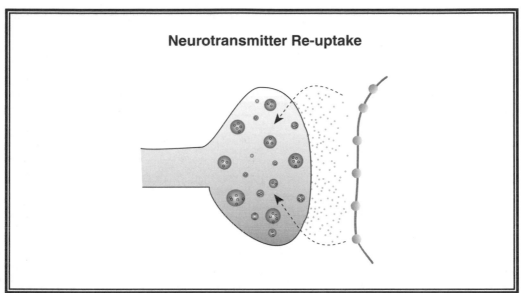

Neurotransmitter Re-uptake

Figure 5-D

Treatment

Treatment with antidepressant medications is described in detail in chapter 14. However, some issues regarding treatment are warranted at this point.

Although atypical depression often presents with unique symptoms, depressions associated with either NE or 5-HT dysfunction look almost identical from a behavioral perspective. Until safe, cost-effective lab tests are available to practitioners, the psychiatrist is faced with an uncertainty regarding the underlying biochemical disorder. Is it NE or 5-HT based? Antidepressants fall into three broad classes: those that target NE dysfunction, 5-HT antidepressants (SSRIs), and MAO inhibitors. (See figure 5-E and chapter 14). Usually the choice of medication used first (if atypical symptoms are not present) is a "shot in the dark"—either an NE or 5-HT antidepressant—and generally is based more on the particular side effect profiles of the various drugs. Presumably, when a 5-HT drug is chosen, if there is little or no benefit after an adequate clinical trial, then the medication is switched to an NE antidepressant.

When the appropriate medication is found, after several weeks of treatment the person begins to notice a reduction in symptoms (especially vegetative symptoms). Under ideal circumstances the depression may be largely resolved within six to eight weeks (although it often takes longer). The clinical improvement is felt to correspond with a normalization of neuronal functioning, that is, normalized re-uptake and a down-regulation of inhibitory receptors. At such time, despite the improved clinical picture, medication discontinuation is *not* advised. At the point of symptomatic improvement, stopping medications has been associated with a very high acute relapse rate (up to 80 percent). Although the medication has returned nerve cells to a more normal state, the cells are unstable and can easily regress if medication is not on board. Thus continued treatment with the antidepressants for at least six months is necessary. Then cautious discontinuation generally results in stable functioning (the acute relapse rate drops to below 10 percent).

Selective Action of Antidepressant Medication

Generic Name	Brand Name	Norepinephrine Effects	Serotonin Effects	Monoamine Oxidase Effects
imipramine	Tofranil	++	+++	0
desipramine	Norpramin	+++++	0	0
amitriptyline	Elavil	+	++++	0
nortriptyline	Aventyl, Pamelor	+++	++	0
protriptyline[a]	Vivactil	++++	+	0
trimipramine[a]	Surmontil	++	++	0
doxepin[a]	Sinequan, Adapin	+++	++	0
maprotiline	Ludiomil	+++++	0	0
amoxapine	Asendin	++++	+	0
venlafaxine	Effexor	++	+++	0
trazodone	Desyrel	0	++++	0
fluoxetine	Prozac	0	+++++	0
paroxetine	Paxil	0	+++++	0
sertraline	Zoloft	0	+++++	0
bupropion[b]	Wellbutrin	±	±	0
phenelzine	Nardil	0	0	+++++
tranylcypromine	Parnate	0	0	+++++
isocarboxazid	Marplan	0	0	+++++

[a] Uncertain, but likely effects
[b] Atypical antidepressant; uncertain effects but likely to be a dopamine and norepinephrine agonist

Figure 5-E

Above and beyond the goal of preventing acute relapse, keep in mind that major depression is often recurring. However, most patients can learn to notice early signs of returning symptoms (which may emerge several years later) and thus can take quick action to reimplement treatment and "nip it in the bud." Relapse prevention is a realistic and important goal for all people being treated for major depression.

The length of medication treatment for dysthymia is not yet well established, but probably requires prolonged treatment. Fortunately, antidepressants have a good track record of safety in long-term use and are not addictive.

Many millions of depressed patients have been helped with antidepressant medications. Clearly, these drugs work—when properly prescribed. However, it is important to underscore that a number of the personal, emotional, and existential issues that make up the experience of a major depression are not magically resolved by antidepressants. Even under ideal circumstances when medications work well, *most* patients must engage in a good deal of soul-searching, mourning, and working-through. The combined approaches of pharmacotherapy and psychotherapy offer the best chance of successful recovery from depression. This has been documented especially in studies investigating the combined use of antidepressants and two forms of psychotherapy especially designed for treating depression: cognitive-behavioral (Beck 1976) and interpersonal psychotherapy (Klerman et al. 1984).

QUICK REFERENCE
When to Refer for Medication Treatment

Event	Symptoms
Grief becomes clinical depression	Early morning awakening Serious weight loss Anhedonia Agitation
Major depression has vegetative symptoms	Sleep disturbance Appetite disturbance Fatigue Decreased sex drive Agitation or psychomotor retardation Anhedonia
Major depression has atypical symptoms	Pronounced fatigue Hypersomnia Increased appetite and weight gain Rejection sensitivity Panic symptoms Reactive dysphoria
Dysthymia presents with sustained symptoms	Low energy Anhedonia
Daily functioning is markedly impaired	
Presence of **severe** suicidal impulses or psychotic symptoms	
Major depression or dysthymia fails to respond to psychotherapy	

6

Bipolar Disorders

The bipolar disorders (historically referred to as manic-depressive illness) are mood disorders characterized by the essential diagnostic feature of mania or hypomania. In general, these disorders follow cyclic patterns of mood, behavior, and thought alterations, alternating between mania or hypomania and depression. These episodic changes are only core features of a variable, heterogeneous group of illnesses. *DSM-IV* classification distinguishes between bipolar I, bipolar II, cyclothymia, and bipolar disorder not otherwise specified. Further diagnostic distinctions are made depending on severity of symptoms and time-course patterns. Pharmacologic treatment of the bipolar disorders is rapidly evolving, with the bulk of useful data having been generated in the last decade.

Differential Diagnosis

Mania rarely occurs as a primary psychiatric condition by itself, so the presence of a manic episode usually leads to a diagnosis of bipolar disorder, even in the absence of a clear depressive history. The manic episode as defined by *DSM-IV* is "a distinct period of abnormally and persistently elevated, expansive, or irritable mood lasting at least one week (or any duration if hospitalization is necessary)." Additionally, manic episodes are defined as mild, moderate, or severe. If severe, psychotic features may be present, but this is not always the case. Associated with this mood disturbance are combinations of racing thoughts, pressured speech, grandiosity, increased activity, engaging in pleasurable activities, distractibility, and decreased need for sleep. If the above patterns are severe enough to impair occupational or social functioning, or to cause hospitalization, a diagnosis of mania is assigned.

A hypomanic episode, defined as lasting at least throughout a four-day period, is marked by an observable change in functioning and disturbance in mood that is uncharacteristic of the individual's usual nondepressed mood and level of functioning. Hypomania is distinguished from mania by the absence of the significant impairment, or hospitalization, described above.

The onset of mania can follow an abrupt or a gradual course. A useful stage-model categorization of acute mania has been described by Carlson and Goodwin (1973), as follows:

Stages of Acute Mania

Stage 1 (corresponds with hypomania):

- Increased psychomotor activity
- Emotional lability
- Euphoria or grandiosity
- Coherent but tangential thinking

Stage 2 (frank mania):

- Increased psychomotor activity
- Heightened emotional lability
- Hostility, anger
- Assaultive or explosive behavior
- Flight of ideas, cognitive disorganization
- Possible grandiose or paranoid delusions

Stage 3 (exhibited by some patients):

- Frenzied psychomotor activity
- Incoherent thought processes
- Ideas of reference, disorientation, delirium
- Florid psychosis (indistinguishable from other psychotic disorders, although usually mood congruent)

Case 13

George M. is a 32-year-old man you saw briefly a number of years ago for several intensive therapy sessions following the death of his mother. You know of no other psychiatric history. His family history is significant for his mother being hospitalized twice with "some sort of mental problem." George was in law school at the time and was not informed of the specifics of his mother's illness. His paternal uncle committed suicide when George was 14.

He is, by his report, in a stable marriage of ten years and has two children. He has must been made a partner in a small, successful law firm. He prides himself in being skilled in various areas, including athletics and music.

George called your office yesterday requesting an appointment to discuss recent feelings of "anxiety and stress." When George arrives at your office he is loud and demands to see you immediately because his "time is so valuable." The receptionist is able to escort him to your office fairly quickly, but not before he has attempted to pass out his business cards to other patients in the waiting room. He appears slightly disheveled, is unshaven, and states that he is "afraid to go to his office today," although will not elaborate further.

During the interview he is unable to remain seated for very long and paces in front of the window. He states the reason for the appointment is for you to "help him straighten a few things out." He specifies that he has been working until 2:00 AM every day for the last week because of an upcoming case. He describes this as the "biggest case in recent history" for which he "will become famous." His speech is pressured, and his thought processes are tangential. When you comment that he smells of alcohol, he admits that he regularly needs "a couple of drinks" a day to bring himself "down." You recognize that George's symptoms may indicate a manic episode, and with some difficulty you persuade him to see one of your psychiatrist colleagues for further evaluation.

Bipolar Disorder Facts

- Lifetime prevalence: 0.4 percent to 1.2 percent (mean 0.5 percent).

- Suicide rate: 22 percent.

- Incidence of psychotic features: 47 to 75 percent

- Ratio of men to women: 1:1.

- 60 to 65 percent of patients have positive family history.

- Over-representation in higher socioeconomic and educational groups.

- First episode is usually mania (60 to 80 percent).

- Average age of onset: 32 years; range is 20 to 40 years.

- Average episodes in a lifetime: 7 to 9.

- Average recovery time for depressed state: 9 weeks.

- Average recovery time for manic state: 5 weeks.

- Average recovery time for mixed state: 14 weeks.

Mania may develop as a consequence of a general medical condition (see figure 6-A) or as a result of pharmacologic treatment (see figure 6-B).

Medical Conditions Associated with Mania

- Central nervous system trauma, for example, post-stroke
- Metabolic disorders such as hyperthyroidism
- Infectious diseases such as encephalitis
- Seizure disorders
- Central nervous system tumor

Figure 6-A

Bipolar I Disorder

One or more manic or hypomanic episodes with one or more major depressive episodes generally constitute the diagnosis of bipolar I disorder. Depending on the current presentation, bipolar disorder is subclassified as one of the following (*DSM-IV*):

Bipolar I Subclasses

- Single manic episode—only one manic episode, no previous major depressive episodes.

- Most recent episode hypomanic—current (or most recent) episode hypomanic with at least one previous manic episode.

- Most recent episode manic—current (or most recent) episode manic with either at least one previous major depressive episode or at least one previous manic or hypomanic episode.

- Most recent episode mixed—current (or most recent) episode of at least one week's duration and criteria for both major depressive episode and manic episode are met on a daily basis. Also at least one previous episode of major depression or one previous episode of mania or hypomania.

- Most recent episode depressed—current (or most recent) episode is major depressive and at least one previous manic episode.

- Most recent episode unspecified—current (or most recent) episode meets criteria for major depression, mania, or hypomania (except for duration), with significant distress or functional impairment. Also at least one previous manic episode.

Depression in bipolar disorder meets diagnostic criteria for major depression, with the exceptions of shorter duration and increased frequency. Between episodes, most bipolar patients are relatively asymptomatic, although many will experience symptoms significant enough to interfere with adequate functioning. With increasing age episodes become more frequent and prolonged.

Bipolar II Disorder

Bipolar II disorder is defined as one or more depressive episodes and at least one episode of hypomania. It has been postulated that bipolar II is difficult to differentiate from major depression, for several reasons. First, many patients subjectively do not recognize periods of elevated mood as dysfunctional—or may even deny the existence of such periods because of the predominate depressive element. Second, the patient may primarily manifest irritability rather than classic mood and behavior symptoms of hypomania. Finally, there is considerable variation between individual clinicians' ability to reliably assess for hypomania.

Drugs That Can Induce Mania

- Stimulants (amphetamines)
- Antidepressants (especially tricyclic antidepressants)
- Antihypertensives
- Corticosteroids (prednisone) in higher doses
- Anticholinergics (benztropine, trihexyphenidyl)
- Thyroid hormones (levothyroxine)

Figure 6-B

Case 14

Cheryl R. is a 28-year-old married woman with two children under three years of age. She has been referred by her family doctor, who has been treating her depression for nine months with fluoxetine 20 mg daily. Her physician states that medication adjustment is not indicated and thinks "talking therapy" will be beneficial. Her psychiatric history is negative for hospitalizations, and she has never been in therapy. She describes a "lifetime of sadness" with periodic episodes of suicidal ideation during late adolescence.

Cheryl reports moderate improvement in her depression since starting the medication and wants to continue taking it. However, she says that some of her initial symptoms of irritability, tearfulness, and tiredness have never really improved. She reports continued initial insomnia and describes lying awake worrying about things.

Her major concern is that she is not the "best mother" that she can be. On particularly "bad days" she places the children in front of the television and retreats to her room. She wishes she had more "good days," which occur about every three months and last for about a week. During these periods she begins sewing and crafts projects for the house, socializes with neighbors, exercises, and "feels on top of the world."

She appears slightly nervous and describes her mood as "pretty bad." She describes her marriage as "average" and her children as the "center of her life." She is moderately impatient with the interview questions relative to history taking, since she wants to "get on with things."

You are encouraged by Cheryl's motivation for treatment. However, you internally question whether she may fit the profile for bipolar II. In the process of the diagnostic interview, you elicit enough information indicative of hypomanic periods that predated the initiation of fluoxetine to warrant further consultation with her original prescriber or a psychiatrist.

Cyclothymia

The features of cyclothymia include periods of alternating depression and elation, of at least two years' duration, that do not meet criteria for either major depression or mania (see figure 6-C). During this two-year period, symptoms are never absent for more than two months. Social and occupational impairment may occur during the depressive phase, but typically not during the hypomanic period. However, for many individuals the pervasive, irregular pattern of mood lability eventually affects personal and work relationships. Because "mood swings" are a frequent complaint of individuals with certain personality disorders, it is important to identify the presence of the associated behavioral criteria for hypomania or depression before establishing a diagnosis of cyclothymia.

This is a chronic disorder, with approximately one-third of individuals later developing a major affective disorder (Akiskal et al., cited by Hirschfeld and Goodwin

1988). Cyclothymia is so strikingly consistent with bipolar disorder with regard to symptoms, family history, course, and treatment response, that some clinicians argue for its categorization as a variant of bipolar disorder.

While the "classic" manic is readily diagnosed, differentiating between diagnostic subtypes may be more difficult, especially when a seasonal pattern exists. Further disorders to rule out in the differential diagnosis include attention deficit hyperactivity disorder, schizophrenia, and schizoaffective disorder.

Cyclothymia Criteria

- History of numerous hypomanic and depressive episodes
- The intensity of episodes does not warrant a diagnosis of major depression or full-blown mania
- Not due to any established organic factors or substance abuse

Figure 6-C

Bipolar Disorder Not Otherwise Specified

Disorders with bipolar features which do not meet any specific bipolar disorder criteria fall into this category. *DSM-IV* provides examples of recurring hypomania without major depression symptomatology, mania superimposed on certain delusional or psychotic disorders, or situations in which bipolar disorder which cannot be determined as primary or secondary to medical conditions or substances.

Course Specifiers

Course specifiers for bipolar I or bipolar II disorder are as follows:
- With rapid cycling
- With seasonal pattern—demonstrated temporal relationship between onset of symptoms and time of the year
- With postpartum onset—must be within four weeks postpartum

Rapid cycling bipolar disorder warrants special attention, due to the diagnostic and treatment challenges it presents. Rapid cycling is defined as at least four episodes of either mania, hypomania, or major depression in the previous twelve months. The characteristics of rapid cycling are these:

Rapid Cycling Bipolar Disorder

- Estimated incidence: 10 to 20 percent of bipolar patients
- Poor lithium response
- More common in women, especially postpartum and postmenopausal
- Subclassified as early onset (initial rapid cycling) and late onset (change from "regular" to rapid cycles)

Etiology

Even though manic-depressive illness was first described by Kraepelin in 1921, causational and treatment questions persist. The introduction of lithium as an effective treatment in the 1970s sparked renewed research interest. Yet the complexity and expense of studying this disorder places limits on achieving consistent and replicable data. Proposed etiological theories of bipolar disorder focus more on neurobiology and genetic transmission than on environmental influences, although the latter is not without importance. Unlike the biologic theories discussed in some other chapters of the book, at this time the precise neurochemical dysfunction in bipolar disorder is not clearly established. However, a number of researchers have posed various theories, summarized below:

- J. Rosenthal et al.'s (1986) dysregulation theory includes (but by definition is not specific to) bipolar disorder. In this model, mood is regulated by several homeostatic mechanisms. The failure of a component part leads to the expression of mood outside of set limits, which are identified as the "symptoms" of mania and depression. R. Post, S. Weiss, and O. Chuang (1992) offer a similar explanation: that overactivity in either of the mediating "circuits" of mania or depression leads to the appearance of associated behavioral manifestations.

- The chaotic attractor theory of J. P. Crutchfield et al. (1986) is intriguing and may help explain the unpredictable course of bipolar disorder. This model is predicated on a biochemical defect leading to dysregulation of neurotransmitter synthesis. The type of dysregulation is consistent, but the symptom presentation (either mania or depression) depends on the physiological or environmental conditions at the moment.

- J. C. Ballenger's and R. M. Post's (1980) kindling model of mood disorder is not completely adequate, but it has provided some valuable contributions to the reconceptualization of several psychiatric disorders. This hypothesis states that some psychiatric symptoms are the result of cumulative subclinical biochemical changes in the limbic system. This progressive buildup causes neurons to become more excitable until, eventually, clinically observable symptoms appear.

- Current research, seeking to refine earlier studies, is focusing on secondary neurotransmitter systems, peripheral and central benzodiazepine receptors, the recently isolated dopamine-3 subtype receptor, GABA receptors and subtypes, and ion channels for sodium, potassium, and calcium. Data from collective studies is overwhelming, yet researchers appear to be slowly uncovering findings that are consistent and interwoven.

- Family studies support a high risk-factor association for first-degree relatives with bipolar disorder. Additionally, other conditions are highly represented in relatives of bipolar individuals, including bipolar II, major depression, cyclothymia, schizoaffective disorder, and suicide.

- Twin studies reviewed by Tsuang and Faraone (1990), demonstrate a concordance rate for monozygotic pairs of 58 to 74 percent and for same-sex dizygotic pairs of 17 to 29 percent. From these studies, the importance of shared environmental factors in bipolar disorder was also elucidated.

- Several studies have attempted to identify genetic transmission through a specific gene on the X-chromosome. Although results are inconsistent, this may be the link for certain subsets of patients whose families show no male-to-male transmission and present with early onset (Baron et al. 1987).

In summary, these various theories, although focusing on different aspects of neurobiology, tend to support a strong biological base for bipolar disorder. Probably the most convincing evidence in favor of a biologic etiology remain the relatively good response to pharmacotherapy and the extremely poor response to purely psychological interventions.

Treatment

The evidence is so strongly compelling that bipolar is largely a biologic-based disorder that pharmacologic intervention is the mainstay of treatment. The details of treatment with various pharmacologic agents are discussed in chapter 15.

Although medications are the primary treatment modality for bipolar disorder, it is important to consider the impact of medications in conjunction with other forms of treatment. For instance, milieu therapy, when inpatient care is necessary, will be most effective after initial medication response has reestablished some degree of cooperation and insight. Psychotherapy, especially cognitive, behavioral, and psychoeducational approaches, is effective with the medication-stabilized patient. Group therapy, which can include families, will often revolve around acceptance of the disease as well as of the need for long-term medication treatment, the side effects, and the implications of noncompliance. In instances of medication resistance or contraindications, ECT should be considered.

QUICK REFERENCE
When to Refer for Medication Treatment

Event	Symptoms
Mood indicates mania or hypomania	Expansiveness Overconfidence Euphoria Irritability Labile mood
Mood indicates depression	Criteria for major depression is met (see chapter 5)
Mood indicates mixed state	Coexistence of above
Thought process and judgment become impaired	Lack of insight Flight of ideas Grandiosity Tangentiality Paranoia Delusions Hallucinations
Behavior becomes inappropriate	Pressured speech Psychomotor hyperactivity Decreased need for sleep Hypersexual or promiscuous Increased spending Gambling

7

Anxiety Disorders

Anxiety disorders encompass a broad, heterogeneous group of psychiatric problems. Like depression, anxiety disorders have multiple etiologies. Some appear to be clearly related to biochemical abnormalities, while others are psychogenic in origin. And treatments vary considerably depending on the diagnosis and presumed underlying pathophysiology. Anxiety disorders have often been erroneously seen as mild or benign disorders. However, recent clinical and epidemiological studies indicate that anxiety disorders are quite common—more common even than depression—and exact a heavy toll on individuals and society alike. The current view sees anxiety disorders as often serious, chronic mental illnesses. Especially in severe cases, such as panic disorder, suicide rates are high; alcohol abuse rates reach 30 percent or more; medical services are inappropriately overutilized; and the cardiac-death rate is higher than average.

Differential Diagnosis

Before outlining the main features of each anxiety disorder, it is necessary to define two terms: *panic attacks* and *anxiety symptoms*. Panic attacks are very brief but extremely intense surges of anxiety. The major differences between a panic attack and more generalized anxiety symptoms are differences in the onset, duration, and intensity (see figure 7-A). Panic attacks often "come out of the blue"; that is, they are not necessarily provoked by stress. They come on suddenly, are *extremely* intense, and last anywhere from 1 to 30 minutes and then subside. The patient feels as if he or she will actually die or go crazy as we are not talking about uneasiness but full-blown panic.

The person may continue to feel nervous or upset for several hours, but the attack itself lasts only a matter of minutes. If a patient says, "I've had a continuous panic attack for the past three days," he or she may be having intense anxiety symptoms, but not a true panic attack. In anxiety disorders without panic attacks, the anxiety symptoms can be very unpleasant, but are much less intense; they also can be prolonged or generalized—that is, present most of the day and lasting from days to years. The symptoms of anxiety are as follows:

Symptoms of Anxiety

- Trembling, feeling shaky, restlessness, muscle tension
- Shortness of breath, smothering sensation
- Tachycardia (rapid heartbeat)
- Sweating and cold hands and feet
- Lightheadedness and dizziness
- Paresthesias (tingling of the skin)
- Diarrhea, frequent urination, or both
- Feelings of unreality (derealization)
- Initial insomnia (difficulty falling asleep)
- Impaired attention and concentration
- Nervousness, edginess, or tension

The distinction between anxiety and panic is very important when it comes to making an accurate diagnosis and choosing appropriate treatments.

Although *DSM-IV* includes twelve types of anxiety disorders, the list of disorders in this chapter is somewhat more brief. Patients suffering from post-traumatic stress disorder (PTSD) and a related disorder, acute stress disorder often do present with a host of anxiety symptoms; however, anxiety is but one aspect of PTSD. This syndrome also often includes symptoms of depression, transient psychosis, and dissociation. Thus, we have chosen not to address it here, but in a separate chapter (see chapter 10). Additionally, although obsessive-compulsive disorder (OCD) is considered to be an anxiety disorder, its pathophysiology and treatment varies enough from the anxiety disorders to warrant a separate chapter (see chapter 8).

Anxiety Symptoms Versus Panic Attacks

	Anxiety	Panic
Onset	Can be gradual	Very sudden
Duration	Prolonged	1 to 30 minutes
Intensity	Mild to moderate	Severe
Precipitated by stressors	Generally	Often not

Figure 7-A

Ten anxiety syndromes can be distinguished, as follows:

- Generalized anxiety disorder (GAD)
- Anxiety associated with psychological stress (adjustment disorder with anxiety)
- Specific phobias
- Social phobias
- Agoraphobia without panic
- Anxiety symptoms due to a general medical condition
- Substance-induced anxiety disorder
- Anxiety symptoms secondary to a primary mental disorder
- "Neurotic" anxiety
- Panic disorder

> **Anxiety Facts**
>
> - Lifetime prevalence rates for anxiety disorders: 25 percent.
> - Thirty-seven million people per year suffer from anxiety disorders in the United States.
> - Panic disorder patients are eighteen times more likely to make suicide attempts than normal controls.
> - Incidence of anxiety disorders, women to men: 2:1.
> - It is estimated that only 30 percent of patients with panic disorder receive treatment. Yet treatment is effective in 70 to 90 percent of those so afflicted.

Generalized anxiety disorder

Generalized anxiety disorder is characterized by chronic, low-level anxiety (without panic attacks). Patients with this disorder may have no specific current stressors. Life in general is stressful for them. Such people are often high strung and are chronic worriers.

Anxiety associated with acute psychological stressors

In such disorders, anxiety symptoms are not evident prior to the onslaught of stressors; preclinically the person functions well. Symptoms emerge in the wake of acute life stress.

Specific phobias

These phobias involve fears of specific objects, such as dogs, or places, such as heights. Anxiety is seen only in the phobic situation.

Social phobias

Social phobias involve serious anxiety symptoms experienced only when the person is in social or interpersonal settings, such as speaking before a group, participating in a social gathering, or asking someone for a date.

Agoraphobia without panic

This disorder is characterized by intense fears of being in situations or places from which escape might be difficult or embarrassing. As in other phobias, the anxiety is accompanied by a strong tendency to avoid being in such feared places. Agoraphobia commonly develops in the course of panic disorder, but in agoraphobia without panic, there is no history of full-blown *spontaneous* panic attacks (see "Panic disorder," below). Experiences of anxiety are always associated either with entry into a feared place or situation such as entering a crowded store or with anticipation of such an event.

Anxiety symptoms due to general medical conditions, substance use or abuse, or another primary psychiatric disorder

In these disorders, the anxiety symptoms are secondary to another etiology.

Neurotic anxiety

Neurotic anxiety arises when an individual is beset by significant emotional issues or conflicts but maintains tight defenses against awareness of these inner issues. In other words, the conflicts are unconscious, and what one sees overtly are anxiety symptoms—often "generalized" and *sometimes* in the form of occasional panic attacks. Another version of neurotic anxiety is seen in individuals who are plagued by more conscious conflicts. Often such conflicts take the form of approach-avoidance, such as the person very much wanting to do something but worrying about offending others or violating certain internalized rules or "shoulds." The person feels inwardly torn and will often experience feelings of generalized anxiety.

Panic disorder

Panic disorder is characterized by recurring, intense panic attacks. Many times these attacks appear to be spontaneous, not provoked by identifiable stressors. As the disorder progresses, most patients begin to develop considerable anticipatory anxiety (a rather continuous, mild-to-moderate generalized anxiety as they come to worry when the next attack will occur)—and phobias (agoraphobia is especially common). With time, alcohol abuse and depression commonly develop.

Since the etiology and treatment of these anxiety syndromes vary significantly, each is discussed separately below, with greater detail provided for the disorders that are felt to be more strongly biologically based.

Etiology

For decades, the psychoanalytic theory of neurosis rested on Freud's fundamental notions of the psychogenic origin of anxiety (Freud's second, or revised, theory of anxiety, 1923). Most neurotic disorders were felt to arise from the unconscious perception of danger: realistic anxiety (danger from the environment), moral anxiety (danger from the superego), and id anxiety (danger from the id). Such unconscious judgments involving potential danger provoked "signal anxiety" and ignited defensive operations. When defenses failed, patients experienced manifest anxiety symptoms.

Other dominant psychological views of anxiety have been proposed by cognitive theorists such as Beck. The cognitive model suggests that anxiety is generated when people overevaluate the danger in certain situations or underestimate their coping ability. The perception of danger and loss of control can provoke fight-or-flight responses even in nondangerous circumstances. With anxious people, their perceptions of reality are skewed such that there are many misperceptions and "false alarms."

These psychological theories are not at all incompatible with biologic ones, though they were developed before the physiology of anxiety was well understood.

Biologic Theories

Let's now explore theories of biologic etiology. "Hard-wired" into the nervous system of humans and many animals is a complex network of nerve pathways, brain structures, and glands that are responsible for eliciting the fight-or-flight response. This response triggers a multilevel neurochemical and hormonal reaction designed to mobilize the body and mind during times of potential danger. Nonessential physiological processes shut down (such as digestion, reproduction), and energy is channeled into a host of bodily functions preparing the organism for rapid action. The nervous system also shifts into a state of hyperarousal and vigilance. All of these changes, which occur rapidly and automatically, have evolved to assure survival when a person or animal confronts actual danger situations. Thus, fundamentally, the biologic mechanisms and processes underlying the fight-or-flight response are necessary and adaptive.

The basic components of the fight-or-flight mechanism are depicted schematically in figure 7-B. As stressful events are perceived at the level of the cortex, lower brain areas become activated. In a sense, the limbic system is put on alert. Should ongoing perception result in a conclusion that there is imminent danger, a burst of excitation emanates from a cluster of nerve cell bodies in the brain stem called the locus coeruleus (LC). The LC has sometimes been called the adrenal gland of the brain. The LC nerve cells, which project to the limbic system, are mediated by the neurotransmitter norepinephrine.

The limbic system and adjacent hypothalamus shift into high gear, and by way of the pituitary gland (and other downstream endocrine glands) and the autonomic nervous system, a multitude of stress hormones are released into the system. The brain and body alike are ready for action.

It is also important to discuss yet another feature of the nervous system that plays a role in anxiety. On the surface of about 40 percent of nerve cells in the brain (including cells in the LC) are tiny gateways referred to as chloride ion channels (see figure 7-C). Chloride ions, which carry a slight negative charge, are in abundance in the fluid surrounding nerve cells. The ion channel can be activated (opened) when

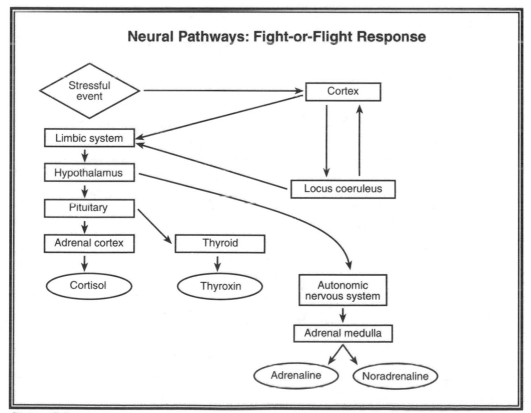

Figure 7-B

stimulated by the naturally occurring neurochemical gamma-aminobutyric acid, GABA for short (see figure 7-C, 2).

As the gate opens, the chloride ions are drawn in. When the nerve cell is infused with negative ions, its electrical characteristics are altered, resulting in decreased excitability; that is, the cell relaxes. This operates as a sort of biological braking mechanism, serving to dampen "limbic alert" and calm overall brain excitation. Benzodiazepine molecules (the substances found in antianxiety medications) also bind to the chloride ion channels, further enhancing the in-flow of negative ions and thus producing a widespread calming in many areas of the brain (see figure 7-C, 3).

This model provides an understanding of the mechanism of action of anti-anxiety medications. It also has led to a theory that may explain some anxiety disorders. Since there is a receptor on the chloride ion channel that responds to benzodiazepine molecules, there is speculation that an endogenous benzodiazepine-like chemical may exist in the CNS. To date, however, such a chemical has yet to be identified. (Although some researchers believe that adenosine may be the chemical.) However, should this theory hold to be true, it may provide an explanation for why some individuals are more "high-strung" and less able to stay calm during stressful times, and why others experience chronic, generalized anxiety. Such individuals *may* suffer from a deficiency of this yet-to-be-identified endogenous neurochemical.

With these biological models in mind, let's begin to look at specific anxiety disorders, many of which represent some type of malfunction in this otherwise-adaptive physiological system.

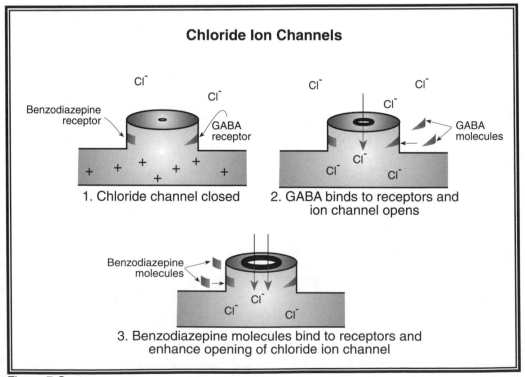

Chloride Ion Channels

1. Chloride channel closed

2. GABA binds to receptors and ion channel opens

3. Benzodiazepine molecules bind to receptors and enhance opening of chloride ion channel

Figure 7-C

Generalized anxiety disorder and anxiety associated with acute stress

In GAD the individual is almost continuously predicting, anticipating, or imagining "dangerous" (unpleasant) events. The limbic system is kept in a perpetual state of alert—on guard for a multitude of "what-ifs." Since daily life rarely presents GAD patients with severely traumatic or life-threatening events, the level of activation does not reach the intensity of threshold of full-blown fight-or-flight. The result is a low-grade, but chronic, state of anxiety.

GAD is primarily felt to be a psychogenic disorder. However, there is some speculation that at least some GAD patients may suffer from a biologically mediated disorder. One hypothesis is that mentioned above: a deficiency of neurochemicals. Another model has emerged more recently. Treatment with serotonin agonists such as buspirone and 5-HT antidepressants has been shown to reduce "what-ifing" (worry) in some GAD patients. However, the mechanism of action and underlying pathophysiology are not well understood.

In stress-induced anxiety disorders, actual psychological stressors have evoked another version of ongoing limbic alert. And in the wake of severe stress, such patients often can have *occasional* full-blown panic attacks. These disorders emerge in response to life-threatening stressors (natural disasters, combat, assaults, automobile accidents) and in response to a host of emotional stressors (loss of a job, serious illness in a relative, marital separation). In many cases, the anxiety symptoms can be seen as normal responses; (that is, they are not pathological). However, the symptoms can be severe enough to warrant treatment.

With GAD and stress-related anxiety, in all likelihood the basic neurobiology is not grossly abnormal. Rather, real or imagined stresses are provoking psychological reactions—which, of course ultimately are biologically mediated.

Specific phobias

Phobias such as the fear of snakes, closed-in spaces, heights, and so on, are generally considered to be associated either with age-appropriate fears (fears that subside with maturation) or conditioned responses. There is little evidence that these disorders are due to biological dysfunction, and medication treatment is generally not warranted.

Social phobias

Social phobias are certainly influenced by developmental and other life experiences (such as the quality of early attachments, the development of appropriate social skills, and adequate experience interacting with others). At the same time, there is rather compelling evidence suggesting that social phobics (and their more pervasively impaired cousins—avoidant personalities) may have a biologically based disorder.

Animal studies have shown that when baby animals are separated from their parents, they typically enter a state of high arousal and agitation—frequently producing some form of vocal distress signal. This is obviously the case with human infants as well. Separation stresses appear to elicit extremely high levels of neuronal activity in the locus coeruleus. One hypothesis holds that this brain area, in addition to its role in evoking fight-or-flight responses, may be a key brain structure designed to trigger arousal and distress behavior in infants separated from caregivers. Presumably, with psychological development and (probably) neurologic maturation, the threshold of LC activity gradually raises. Behaviorally, we see an increased capacity to tolerate separation as children and young animals mature.

What does this have to do with social phobias? One view is that the underlying fear in many social phobias is that the person will be embarrassed, humiliated, and ultimately rejected, which is equivalent to separation. This fear of rejection is also seen in avoidant personalities, so-called hysteroid-dysphorics (see chapter 5), and many people suffering from borderline personality disorders. Animals treated with heterocyclic antidepressants and MAO inhibitors (drugs shown to reduce excitation in the LC) exhibit markedly decreased distress in the face of separation stresses. And during the past decade, clinical trials with antidepressants and MAO inhibitors have shown improvement in broad groups of patients with social phobias and rejection sensitivity. The theory contends that such patients may be chronically experiencing very low thresholds of arousal at the level of the locus coeruleus—accounting for their exquisite sensitivity to humiliation, separation, and rejection.

Agoraphobia without panic

The anxiety experienced with this disorder only occurs when the patient must go into feared situations (such as a store) or in the moments before entering the phobic situation (anticipating anxiety). Although such experiences of anxiety ultimately do involve an activation of the limbic system, the primary disorder is felt to be largely psychogenic, a conditioned fear response. Medications are sometimes used to treat agoraphobia without panic; however, this disorder is not felt to be biologically based.

Anxiety symptoms due to general medical conditions

Certain systemic medical illnesses and primary neurologic disorders can dysregulate CNS neurotransmitters and cause or contribute to anxiety symptoms (see figure 7-D). Note that most anxiety symptoms associated with these medical conditions present in the form of generalized anxiety, generally not panic attacks.

Substance-induced anxiety disorders

A common cause of anxiety symptoms can be traced to drug use or abuse (see figure 7-E).

Medical Disorders Associated with Anxiety

- Adrenal tumor
- Alcoholism
- Angina pectoris
- Cardiac arrhythmia
- CNS degenerative disease
- Cushing's disease
- Coronary insufficiency
- Delirium[a]
- Hypoglycemia

- Hyperthyroidism
- Ménière's disease (early stages)
- Parathyroid disease
- Partial-complex seizures
- Postconcussion syndrome
- Premenstrual syndrome
- Pulmonary embolism
- Mitral valve prolapse[b]

[a] Delirium can occur as a result of many toxic and metabolic conditions and often produces anxiety and agitation.
[b] The mitral valve prolapse probably does not cause anxiety, but it has been found that MVP and anxiety disorders often coexist. This may be due to some common underlying genetic factor.

Figure 7-D

Drugs That Can Cause Anxiety

- Amphetamines
- Asthma medications
- Caffeine
- CNS depressants (withdrawal from)

- Cocaine
- Nasal decongestants (spray)
- Steroids
- Appetite suppressants

Figure 7-E

Anxiety symptoms secondary to primary psychiatric disorders

Certainly, anxiety symptoms are seen in a very wide range of psychiatric disorders, including schizophrenia, mania, PTSD, agitated depressions, and severe personality disorders. It is important to keep in mind that anxiety *symptoms* do not necessarily signal a diagnosis of anxiety *disorder*. Almost without exception, however, when anxiety is associated with a more primary mental disorder, psychotropic medication treatment is aimed at the primary disorder. (Refer to appropriate chapters for descriptions of etiology and treatment.)

Neurotic anxiety

Although the term *neurosis* has fallen out of favor in some professional circles, the concept still has merit. As conceived of here, neurotic anxiety is a condition in which manifest symptoms of anxiety are evident but the underlying problem can ultimately be traced to unconscious conflicts, or unrecognized inner emotional issues. A common example of this is illustrated in Case 15.

Case 15

Rob S. is 42 and recently lost his wife to breast cancer. Emotionally, he grits his teeth and blocks his inner grief. But the overcontainment of his inner feelings of loss has resulted in a tense, brittle adaptation. Rob feels little sadness, but his heart races, he experiences tension headaches, and he has initial insomnia. The problem does not lie in disordered neurons, but in overdefensiveness; and the solution is not to be found in a pill, but rather in the process of working through and mourning (possibly in the context of psychotherapy). To assume a biological etiology and attempt to medicate away anxiety symptoms with this man would only create more distance between his conscious awareness and his inner painful emotional concerns.

As mentioned earlier, some neurotic conflicts that generate anxiety may also be experienced on a conscious level. But again, these are best seen as psychogenic rather than as biologically rooted problems.

Panic disorder

The biological factors that set the stage for the emergence of panic disorder may arise spontaneously (be truly endogenous) or can be set in motion by major life stressors. One theory holds that major separations, losses, or other disruptions of attachments may sensitize and reactivate the locus coeruleus. Biochemical factors operate to alter cellular functions in the LC, lowering the excitation threshold for those neurons.

Panic disorder begins with the eruption of full-blown panic attacks—many of which (as mentioned earlier) occur "out of the blue" in low- or no-stress situations. Some individuals with panic disorder suffer from relatively infrequent attacks (a few per month); in more severe cases, attacks can occur several times a day and oftentimes even during sleep. The *noradrenergic hypothesis* holds that the intense, recurring attacks are caused by hypersensitive neurons in the LC or a dysfunction in the natural braking mechanism in the LC nerve cells or both (see figure 7-F).

The nerve axon in figure 7-F impinges back on itself and releases its neurotransmitter norepinephrine (also called noradrenaline, hence the term "noradrenergic hypothesis"). The neurotransmitter typically stimulates inhibitory receptors on the

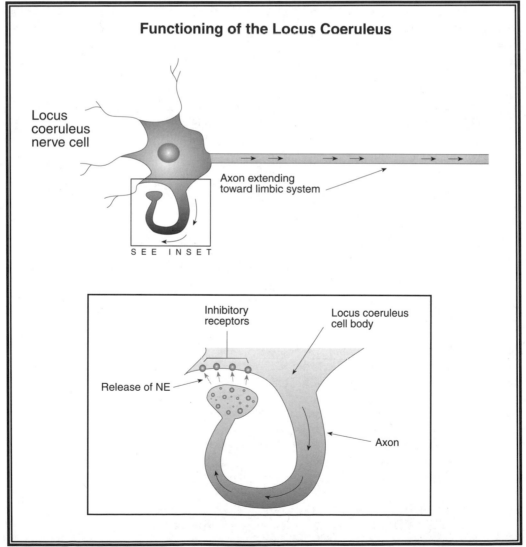

Functioning of the Locus Coeruleus

Locus coeruleus nerve cell

Axon extending toward limbic system

SEE INSET

Inhibitory receptors

Locus coeruleus cell body

Release of NE

Axon

Figure 7-F

cell body, acting to reduce excitability. However, in panic disorder, the inhibitory receptors ("brakes") are felt to be dysfunctional. Once stimulated, the LC cell continues to fire alerting signals to the limbic system, uninhibited by the normal braking mechanism. Antipanic medications (especially antidepressants) are hypothesized to have their effect by normalizing the operation of LC inhibitory receptors (see chapters 14 and 16).

Treatment

Generalized anxiety disorder

For many patients, psychological approaches are the treatment of choice. These techniques include stress management, cognitive-behavioral treatment[1], relaxation training, meditation, and psychotherapy. Also, for GAD patients in good health who do not experience coexisting panic attacks, a program of regular, aerobic-level exercise can be very beneficial. Note that individuals with panic disorder often experience an *exacerbation* of panic attacks when involved in strenuous exercise.

When medication is indicated, the clinician has three choices:

• Benzodiazepines (the class of drugs often termed minor tranquilizers or antianxiety medications) can be used in severe cases of GAD. However, the use of benzodiazepines to treat GAD has been the subject of considerable controversy. Great concern has arisen regarding potential benzodiazepine abuse and dependence. Certainly, people who chronically use benzodiazepines do develop a physiologic dependence on these medications. Nonetheless, concern in the media and medical profession alike may have been overstated. The vast majority of chronically anxious patients do not abuse nor become addicted to these medications and rarely require progressive increases in doses. The individuals who do, in fact, present a significant risk of abuse are people with a personal or family history of alcohol or other substance abuse. With such individuals, benzodiazepines are not appropriate. (Guidelines and cautions regarding treatment appear in chapters 12 and 16.)

• The atypical antianxiety medication buspirone has been used with some success with GAD patients. This medication offers the benefits of reduced rumination and worry, but without the problems of sedation and potential drug dependence seen with benzodiazepines. Buspirone is not addictive and thus provides a treatment option for GAD patients with substance abuse risk.

• Both cyclic and serotonergic antidepressants (SSRIs) are being used increasingly to treat chronically anxious patients. Clinical-anecdotal data is available, although to date few controlled trials have been conducted. (See chapter 14 for information regarding treatment with 5-HT antidepressants.)

Anxiety associated with acute stress

Again, for most individuals, psychological approaches are best suited for treating acute stress reactions. However, antianxiety medications can be an important ad-

---

1. For a review of cognitive-behavioral treatments for anxiety disorders, the reader is referred to *Depression and Anxiety Management*, an audiotape by John Preston, New Harbinger Publications, 1993.

junct to treatment, especially when the patient is experiencing considerable amounts of agitation or insomnia. The classic form of anxiety-related insomnia is initial insomnia (difficulty falling asleep). Middle insomnia or early morning awakening should alert the clinician to a diagnosis of depression. Medications used to treat daytime anxiety include the whole range of benzodiazepines, and for sleep the so-called sedative-hypnotics (see chapter 16). Typically, drug treatment for acute stress is short-term (one to four weeks), in combination with crisis intervention and other psychological treatments.

Specific and social phobias

Specific phobias generally are not treated with psychotropic medications. Social phobias often respond well to cognitive-behavioral treatment. When medications are used, the clinician has two main alternatives: For occasional use—for example to reduce anxiety associated with theatrical performances or public speaking—the beta blocker propranolol has been shown to be quite effective. This drug does little to alter the cognitive aspects of anxiety (worry), but effectively reduces many physiological symptoms such as rapid heart rate. Anxious patients treated with propranolol take the medication only prior to the stressful event, ingesting 20–80 mg about one hour before.

More pervasive forms of social anxiety (and avoidant personality disorder) may be treated with MAO inhibitors or SSRIs (see chapter 14), in addition to psychotherapy and social-skills training.

Agoraphobia without panic

The treatment of choice for this disorder includes psychotherapy, relaxation training, and behavioral treatment (graded exposure to feared situations). Such approaches have a solid track record of effectiveness, and medication treatment as a sole therapy generally is not effective. However, often patients are treated with psychotropic medications in the early phase of graded exposure therapy. Minor tranquilizers (benzodiazepines) and beta blockers (such as propranolol) can be used to somewhat reduce the level of anxiety as the patient begins gradually to reenter anxiety-provoking situations. As the patient starts to experience success and a sense of mastery, the medications can be gradually phased out.

Anxiety symptoms due to general medical conditions, substance abuse, or primary psychiatric disorder

These symptoms usually are not directly treated with psychotropic medications. Rather the primary medical disorder is treated, or the patient is referred for treatment of a chemical dependency problem (see chapter 12). When psychotropics are employed, they generally are used for short periods of time. Medications of choice are the benzodiazepines (although they should be used with extreme caution in patients with a substance abuse disorder).

As noted earlier, when a primary psychiatric disorder is diagnosed, generally medication treatment targets the primary illness, such as antipsychotics for schizophrenia or antidepressants for agitated depression.

Neurotic anxiety

In neurotic anxiety, medication treatment is generally contraindicated, since the reduction of overt anxiety symptoms can serve to further block awareness of core emotional conflicts. The exceptions are these:

- If the patient has inadequate ego strength to tolerate a more "uncovering" psychological approach.

- If the patient is not psychologically minded or has a low level of cognitive functioning.

- If the clinician must work with a highly symptomatic client in *very* brief therapy.

- If manifest anxiety symptoms are severe. In such cases, short-term treatment with benzodiazepines may help reduce suffering, restore functioning in daily life, and help the patient stabilize. This can then be followed by medication reduction and psychotherapy.

Panic disorder

Panic disorder is the anxiety disorder for which medication treatment plays its most important role. This often-devastating illness is quite responsive to combined medication and psychological treatment. It is helpful to focus on four somewhat discrete aspects of this disorder, each of which requires targeted treatments:

- Panic attacks

- Anticipatory anxiety

- Phobias

- Associated features—alcohol abuse, depression

Panic attacks must be either eliminated or greatly reduced in the initial phase of treatment. Some behavioral and cognitive techniques have been developed to reduce panic attacks, although antipanic medications take effect more rapidly and have a solid track record as safe and highly effective drugs. Antipanic medications fall into three groups:

- High-potency benzodiazepines, such as alprazolam, clonazepam

- Antidepressants (tricyclics and SSRIs)[2]

- MAO inhibitors

See chapters 14 and 16 for more on these types of medications.

The first goal of treatment is to stop or reduce attacks. However, even when this is successful, anticipatory anxiety and phobias can, and often do, continue unabated. Thus, the second step is to reduce anticipatory anxiety and phobic avoidance using behavioral techniques, especially graded exposure and desensitization (see Preston 1993). These techniques are highly effective, but only after there is good containment of panic symptoms.

Often, especially in more chronic cases, major depression, alcohol abuse, dependency, or both develop along with primary panic symptoms. In that event, appropriate antidepressant medication treatment and/or involvement in Alcoholics Anonymous or a chemical-dependency treatment program becomes necessary.

---

2. To date, all antidepressants have been shown to reduce panic symptoms, with one exception: bupropion. This antidepressant can at times exacerbate panic attacks, and thus should be used with caution.

Finally, when primary anxiety or panic symptoms are resolved, many panic disorder patients often choose to pursue more traditional psychotherapy. As mentioned earlier, a number of panic patients have encountered major losses and must begin the journey of working through these major life changes. In our experience, however, insight-oriented treatment typically must await the resolution of primary panic symptoms.

Unfortunately a large percentage of patients relapse when medications are discontinued—as many as 70 percent have a return of panic symptoms if medications are withdrawn a year after treatment is initiated. Panic disorder, thus, appears to be an often chronic condition. To date, there are no very long-term follow-up studies tracking the course of this disorder. However, for practical purposes, the clinician should anticipate medication treatment lasting at least one year. Then a trial discontinuation or medication reduction can be implemented to determine if continued treatment is necessary.

QUICK REFERENCE
When to Refer for Medication Treatment

The following anxiety disorders generally are *not* treated with psychotropic medications; a referral should be made only if the patient's symptoms are severe or fail to respond to psychological treatments:

- Generalized anxiety disorder
- Specific phobias
- Social phobias
- Agoraphobia without panic

If anxiety symptoms occur in the context of:

- A general medical condition
- Substance use or abuse
- Another primary psychiatric disorder

Then treat the primary disorder.

Psychotherapy is the treatment of choice for:

- Anxiety associated with acute stress
- Neurotic anxiety

Treat the following symptoms with medications only if symptoms are severe and fail to respond to psychological treatment:

- Initial insomnia
- Daytime agitation or restlessness
- Impaired concentration

Treatment with medication should be short term (1-4 weeks).

A combination of medication and psychological therapy is the treatment of choice for panic disorder, as demonstrated by the following:

Event	Symptom
Recurring panic attacks	Sudden onset Intense anxiety Short duration (1-30 minutes) Some attacks are spontaneous
Patient has had four or more attacks in past month	
Patient has developed significant anticipatory anxiety, phobias, avoidance	
Patient has developed secondary symptoms	Clinical depression Alcohol abuse

8

Obsessive-Compulsive Disorder

Obsessive-compulsive disorder (OCD) until recently was considered to be a very rare disorder. However, newer epidemiological studies show OCD to be just as common as panic disorder, and two to three times as common as schizophrenia or bipolar disorder.

OCD is a chronic psychiatric condition, often first emerging in childhood, and potentially lasting a lifetime. It results in considerable emotional suffering. Yet until recent times, few of those afflicted sought treatment. This is probably due to the common tendency for OCD patients to experience humiliation and shame over symptoms that they generally consider to be "crazy" or "irrational" and thus not to seek out professional help.

Differential Diagnosis

The major features of this disorder are recurring obsessions (persistent intrusive, troublesome thoughts or impulses that are recognized by the patient as senseless) and compulsions (repetitive behaviors or rituals enacted in response to an obsession, such as repeatedly checking to see if doors are locked, excessive hand washing, and counting). In order to meet the criteria for obsessive-compulsive disorder, the obsessions and compulsions must create significant distress and be time-consuming enough or otherwise interfere with normal routines, work, activities, or relationships (*DSM-IV*).

Two-thirds of OCD patients are plagued by obsessions regarding dirtiness, contamination, and germs, with corresponding compulsions such as cleaning and hand washing. Another 20 percent primarily are worried about safety issues and engage

Obsessive-Compulsive Disorder Facts

- Lifetime prevalence: 2.5 percent.

- Ratio of men to women: 1:1.

- Age of onset: Although many cases of OCD begin in adolescence or early adulthood, about half begin in childhood. The incidence of OCD in children is 1 to 1.5 percent.

- Course: Although some milder cases of OCD can be transient, most moderate-to-severe cases last for many years if untreated.

in repetitive checking rituals (checking to see if doors are locked, if the stove is turned off, retracing their route when driving to make sure they have not accidentally hit a pedestrian). The remaining patients are concerned with a sense of incompleteness, or lack of order or symmetry, and engage in rituals designed to make their environment "just right." At the heart of most obsessions and compulsions are two key elements: excessive self-doubt and intense worry regarding the safety of oneself and others. In addition to OCD symptoms, which are a tremendous source of suffering in their own right, two-thirds of OCD patients also experience episodes of major depression.

Many people will experience occasional obsessions and compulsions, especially when under stress or when they sense some loss of control over the environment or inner emotions. These more minor, transient obsessions and compulsions do not constitute OCD, which in contrast is a chronic and often incapacitating disorder.

Some similarities exist between OCD and obsessive-compulsive personality disorder (OCP); however, there are notable differences. For treatment purposes, it is important to distinguish between OCD and OCP. With OCD the person feels "under attack" by the obsessions and compulsive rituals; the symptoms are quite painful and ego-dystonic. In contrast, OCP traits (perfectionism, stinginess, emotional rigidity, over-devotion to work) are experienced as a part of oneself, or ego-syntonic.

Some patients are described as suffering from impulse-control disorders (ICD): gambling, overeating, and so on. Although OCD patients subjectively feel "seized" by an impulse to carry out rituals, notable differences exist between OCD and true ICDs. Those experiencing impulse-control problems find the actions, such as overeating, to be pleasurable. In contrast, OCD patients never enjoy carrying out rituals (beyond *some* reduction in anxiety). Also, impulse-control patients rarely are riddled with self-doubt or worries about harming others—again in sharp contrast to OCD. Finally, the medication treatments successful in OCD (described below) have not been shown to be helpful in various forms of impulse-control disorder.

Anorectics often exhibit a host of obsessions and compulsions (regarding eating—sizes and portions, times for meals, body weight)—yet two notable differences exist between anorectics and OCD patients. Obsessive-compulsive disorder patients almost always admit that the worries and rituals are irrational, whereas most anorectics don't appreciate the irrationality of their acts. Also, medications found to be effective for OCD generally are not effective in the treatment of anorexia nervosa.

Etiology

Traditional psychoanalytic theories posited psychogenic theories for what was once called obsessive-compulsive neurosis. These primarily involved early developmental experiences with perfectionistic, overly strict, and rigid parents who imposed unrealistic standards and stifled the child's emerging autonomy. These theories likely do apply to the development of OCP, but not necessarily OCD. In recent years a number of findings from clinical practice and neurobiology have convincingly argued a biological basis for OCD. Let's take a look at some of this evidence.

The disorder emerges early, often in late childhood, and maintains remarkable symptomatic stability throughout life. The incidence in the general population is 2.5 percent, yet it is 7 percent in first-degree relatives, suggesting a possible genetic loading for the disorder. Also, diseases such as certain types of encephalitis, that selectively damage areas of the basal ganglia (subcortical brain structures) have been shown to result in OCD-symptoms.

Probably most convincing are the findings from pharmacological and neuro-imaging studies. A very large number of clinical studies have shown that OCD patients can be helped by treatment with 5-HT antidepressants. And this holds true even in OCD patients without coexisting depression. In addition, antidepressants that do not affect serotonin are not effective in alleviating OCD symptoms. The 5-HT antidepressants selectively increase serotonin activity in the brain and probably more specifically in the basal ganglia, cingulate gyrus, and prefrontal cortex.

Finally, several studies of brain metabolic functioning reveal that in highly symptomatic OCD patients there is a significant increase in metabolic activity (thus increased activation) in the prefrontal cortex and basal ganglia. Furthermore, this abnormal metabolic activity becomes normalized when patients are treated with 5-HT antidepressants. (Baxter et al. 1992; Rapoport 1991).

Two theories have emerged from these data. The first is that the frontal lobes normally act to inhibit or override the emergence of primitive instinctual urges. However, in OCD this inhibition fails, and we see the eruption of innate urges, or behavioral routines such as nest building, grooming, and the checking of territorial boundaries—instinctual behaviors associated with more primitive species. In this model, ordering, straightening, cleaning, hand washing, checking door locks, and so forth, may reflect human versions of a breakthrough of these more primitive urges.

A second theory holds that there are naturally existing neural pathways that typically serve adaptive purposes, especially when people are exposed to potentially dangerous situations. The frontal cortex serves as the launching site for worry. When exposed to dangerous stimuli, the frontal lobes guide and direct sustained perceptual focus and attention. In essence, arousal is passed through a feedback circuit (see figure 8-A). In normal individuals this serves to maintain alertness and vigilance until

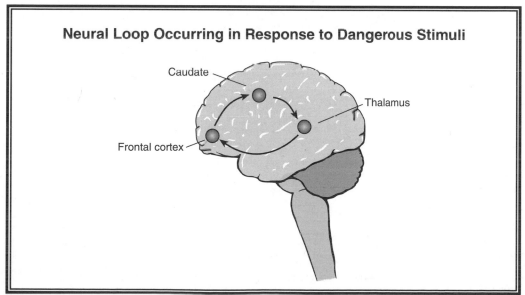

Neural Loop Occurring in Response to Dangerous Stimuli

Caudate

Thalamus

Frontal cortex

Figure 8-A

it is determined that there is no danger; then the inner reverberating loop shuts down. Presumably, this neural loop fails to inhibit itself in OCD. The brain continues to sense danger (or to "worry" about danger) despite cognitive evidence to the contrary. The patient gets caught in an ongoing repetition of worry and engages in behavioral attempts to reduce the worry (the rituals). The caudate is richly innervated by 5-HT neurons. When these nerve cells are activated by 5-HT antidepressants, the inhibitory serotonegic cells reduce the excessive metabolic activity, shut down the maladaptive loop, and OCD symptoms diminish.

Treatment

Standard psychotherapy is notoriously ineffective with OCD. To date, two approaches to treatment are, however, proving to be helpful in reducing symptoms in this truly devastating mental illness.

The first are behavioral techniques: exposure and response prevention. Exposure amounts to systematic, gradual exposure to anxiety-provoking stimuli, for example, for a patient afraid of contamination by germs, the exposure trial might involve having the patient clean a toilet without using gloves. Response prevention amounts to helping the patient avoid rituals, such as avoiding hand washing. The rituals, if carried out, usually reduce anxiety. With response prevention, the initial experience is that the patient will encounter considerable anxiety as he or she avoids the ritualistic behavior. Yet, with repeated exposures or response prevention, gradually the anxiety diminishes. This is an emotionally difficult treatment to embark upon, but is one shown to be successful in 65 to 75 percent of patients—given an adequate number of trials, typically 20 to 25 sessions.

Medication treatment has become more successful with the advent of selective 5-HT antidepressants. These medications, as noted earlier, are given to OCD patients even if they are not clinically depressed. In addition to their antidepressant effects, these drugs reduce OCD symptoms directly. Treatment with medications for OCD *generally* requires doses higher than those used to treat clinical depression (see figure 8-B). Aside from higher doses, treatment guidelines are the same as for treating depression (see chapter 14).

Psychotropic medications are felt to be effective in 50 to 65 percent of OCD cases. Unfortunately, if patients stop medications, there is a 95 percent relapse rate; thus chronic treatment is necessary. In all likelihood, combined behavioral and pharmacologic treatment offers the best promise for successful outcome.

5-HT Antidepressants Useful in Treating OCD			
Generic Name	Brand Name	Typical Depression Dose (mg/day)	Typical OCD Dose (mg/day)
Clomipramine	Anafranil	150–200	200–300
Fluoxetine	Prozac	20–40	20–80
Sertraline	Zolof	50–150	50–200
Paroxetine	Paxil	20–30	20–50

Figure 8-B

QUICK REFERENCE
When to Refer for Medication Treatment

Event	Symptoms
Persistent symptoms that are ego-dystonic, create significant distress, and/or interfere with normal routines	Obsessions—intrusive, troublesome thoughts or impulses
	Compulsions—repetitive rituals enacted to reduce anxiety generated by obsessions
	Comorbid clinical depression

9

Psychotic Disorders

This chapter deals with the group of disorders referred to as "psychotic disorders." The term *psychotic* is defined in *DSM-IV* as "gross impairment in reality testing and the creation of a new reality." Although a number of symptoms can be seen in the context of psychotic disorders, impaired reality testing is the central defining feature. Impaired reality testing may be seen behaviorally in the form of bizarre behavior. However, it is most clearly observed in patients' verbal output and content of speech; psychotic patients reveal false beliefs (delusions) and seriously impaired perceptions (hallucinations). You will note that the definition involves not only impairment of reality testing, which alone would be only confusion, but also the "creation of a new reality," such as delusions (I am being followed by the FBI) or hallucinations (I hear a voice telling me I am bad).

Psychosis, per se, is not a diagnosis but a symptom. There are a number of types of psychotic disorders, which have traditionally been classified into two broad groups: functional psychoses and organic psychoses. The term *functional* refers to those psychoses with a presumed psychological etiology and *organic* refers to those with a presumed biological etiology. Schizophrenia was traditionally classified as a functional psychosis; however, more recent research findings strongly suggest that schizophrenia has a biological basis; that is, it is an endogenous mental disorder. The distinction appears to still have some utility, however, in that organic psychoses can be seen as those due to an underlying medical disorder or drugs, (for example, psychotic organic brain syndromes, amphetamines), and functional psychoses comprise those with an unclear etiology.

Psychotic Disorder Facts

- 1 percent of the population has schizophrenia.

- 1 to 4 percent of psychiatric admissions have delusional disorder.

- 10 to 15 percent of medical-surgical patients in a general hospital have delirium.

- 15 percent of patients diagnosed with dementia have a treatable condition.

- Delirium is most common in the very young and the elderly.

Differential Diagnosis

Organic Psychoses

The term *organic psychosis* is used for those organic or neurologic conditions that have psychotic symptoms.

In *DSM-IV*, these are divided into:

- Disorders of cognition—delirium, dementia, and amnestic and other cognitive disorders

- Psychotic disorders due to a general medical condition, with delusions or hallucinations

- Mood disorders due to a general medical condition

- Catatonic disorder due to a general medical condition

The term *delirium* refers to a condition with impaired attention and clouding of consciousness. There is marked confusion; thinking is fragmented or disorganized; speech is rambling; and mood is often quite labile. This is sometimes referred to as an acute confusional state. *Dementia* refers to a condition in which there is an impairment in memory and higher cognitive abilities, such as judgment and abstract thinking, but without clouding of consciousness. Typically, in dementia short-term memory is impaired more than long-term. *Amnestic disorder* refers to a condition of selectively impaired memory without other cognitive impairment. Psychotic disorder due to a general medical condition (GMC) takes two forms: with delusions and with hallucinations. Mood disorder due to a GMC has prominent mood symptoms; either manic or depressive. Psychotic disorder due to a GMC, mood disorder due to a GMC, and catatonic disorder due to a GMC share the same features as their counterpart functional disorder (psychotic disorder, manic or depressive disorder, catatonic schizophrenia) but are caused by a medical illness.

The causes of organic psychoses are legion, but may be grouped into the following types:

Causes of Organic Psychoses

- Metabolic

    Organ failure, such as renal failure

    Hypoxia

    Hypoglycemia

    Vitamin deficiency

    Endocrinopathy, such as hyperthyroidism

    Fluid or electrolyte imbalance

    Porphyria

- Drug or alcohol intoxication or withdrawal

- Infections

Causes of Organic Psychoses (*continued*)

- Epilepsy

- Head injury

- Vascular diseases, such as lupus

- Intracranial tumor

- Cerebral degenerative diseases
  Dementia, such as Alzheimer's disease
  Multiple sclerosis
  Huntington's chorea
  Parkinson's disease

Functional Psychoses

The functional psychoses can be divided into the following diagnoses:
- Brief reactive psychosis
- Delusional disorder
- Schizophrenia
- Schizophreniform disorder
- Schizoaffective disorder
- Induced psychotic disorder
- Psychotic disorder not otherwise specified (atypical)
- Major depression with psychotic features
- Bipolar disorder, manic

Brief reactive psychosis refers to a condition in which a person has psychotic symptoms lasting from a few hours to a month. There usually is some identifiable stressor that has precipitated the psychosis, and the person demonstrates significant emotional turmoil. The symptoms may be identical to that seen in schizophrenia, but they remit in a fairly brief period of time (less than one month).

Delusional disorder refers to a disorder with persistent nonbizarre delusions without bizarre behavior or prominent hallucinations. Thus, if someone has the delusion they are under surveillance by the FBI, they may meet the criteria. But if delusions are bizarre—for example, if a patient thinks she is under surveillance by Martians—she does not meet the criteria. The disorder is classified by type of delusion: erotomanic, grandiose, jealous, persecutory, or somatic.

Schizophrenia refers to a disorder of longer than six months' duration with prominent psychotic symptoms. This disorder is discussed in detail below. *Schizophreniform disorder* has the same criteria as schizophrenia, but is of less than six months' duration.

Schizoaffective disorder refers to a condition in which the person has not only schizophrenia but also significant episodes of mood disorder, either manic or depressive.

In *induced psychotic disorder*, the person develops psychosis as a result of an intense relationship and identification with someone who is already psychotic, for example, in folie à deux. Here the person typically has poorly defined self-other boundaries and will begin to mimic psychotic symptoms seen in the other individual. (Psychotic symptoms seen in severe affective disorders and mania and depressive psychoses are covered in chapters 5 and 6.)

Now let's discuss schizophrenia in more detail, using it as the prototype of functional psychosis.

Schizophrenia

Schizophrenia as a syndrome has been recognized for thousands of years. As long ago as the Hippocratic school, a syndrome called dementia (with behaviors and symptoms akin to schizophrenia) was recognized as distinct from "mania" and "melancholia." Kraepelin (1898) described a syndrome he called dementia praecox. This referred to a psychotic disorder with progressive debilitation leading to severe impairment of social and intellectual functioning. In his view, this syndrome was invariably progressive, with a very poor prognosis, although more recent research questions the progressive nature of all schizophrenic disorders.

The clinical picture of schizophrenia varies depending on the particular phase of the disorder. *DSM-IV* divides the course of schizophrenia into three phases: prodromal, active, and residual. During the prodromal phase, patients show a deterioration in their level of functioning, without being actively psychotic. In this phase, the patient may show mostly "negative" symptoms (discussed below), such as isolativeness, blunted or flat affect, and lack of initiative. There may also be a disruption of sleep patterns. In the active phase, the person is floridly psychotic, with disorganized thinking, delusions, and hallucinations. In the following residual phase, the patient continues to be impaired, but without severe psychotic symptoms. Social isolation and peculiar affect and thinking may persist, to a degree.

For a diagnosis of schizophrenia, these three phases must last more than six months and must not be due to a mood disorder. Three types of schizophrenia are delineated: catatonic (prominent movement disorder), disorganized (severe thought disorganization), and paranoid (prominent paranoid delusions with mild disorganization of thinking). Undifferentiated and residual types are categories for those who do not fit the above three types but have a mix of features.

Case 16

George A. was a 19-year-old college student who was brought to the student health clinic by his roommate. It was difficult to get a clear history from George because he kept changing the subject and making odd and disconnected statements. His roommate reported George had been progressively more isolative the past four months. The past month he had been staying up late at night and had become somewhat secretive. He wrote notes to himself in a special notebook and made odd comments about God and Christ and about something "coming soon." His personal hygiene had deteriorated, and he sometimes went several days without bathing or changing clothes.

George reported that he felt that he was on a special mission to prepare for the second coming of Christ and that he sometimes heard God or the devil speaking to him. He thought it was necessary that he die or suffer in order to atone for his sins and the sins of the world. He admitted that he was doing poorly in school, but explained that doing God's work was more important. His roommate, who had known him in high school, described him as quiet, shy, and somewhat of a loner. He had never dated.

George was treated with antipsychotic medication, and the delusions and hallucinations resolved. But he continued to have difficulty in college and eventually dropped out of school and returned home to stay with his family.

This case illustrates the prodromal, active, and residual phases. George A. is described as having a somewhat schizoid premorbid personality, as is classically described (although some studies have shown that this is present in only about 50 percent of those diagnosed with schizophrenia). This case also illustrates what are called positive and negative symptoms. For practical purposes, it is helpful to group schizophrenic symptoms into three categories, as outlined below. (Note that characterological features are not psychotic symptoms per se, but do often accompany the more core positive or negative symptoms.)

Schneiderian First-Rank Symptoms

- *Thought broadcasting*—belief that one's thoughts are escaping aloud into the external world.

- *Experiences of alienation*— belief that one's thoughts, feelings, and actions are not one's own.

- *Experiences of influence*— belief that one's thoughts, feelings, and actions are being controlled by some external agent.

- *Complete auditory hallucinations*—hallucinations of voices coming from outside one's head.

- *Delusional perceptions*— a real, normal perception to which one attaches a private meaning.

Schizophrenia Symptoms

- Positive symptoms:
  - Hallucinations
  - Delusions
  - Agitation
  - Floridly bizarre behavior
  - First-rank symptoms (see sidebar)
- Negative symptoms:
  - Anhedonia
  - Apathy
  - Blunted affect
  - Poverty of thought
  - Feelings of emptiness
  - Amotivational states
- "Characterological" symptoms:
  - Social isolation or alienation
  - Marked feelings of inadequacy
  - Poorly developed social skills

The distinction between positive and negative symptoms appears to be significant because of both their differential responses to medication and their differing clinical course and probable differing etiology.

Traditionally, as mentioned above, schizophrenia was seen as being like dementia praecox—as having a chronic, progressive course. More recent research has called this into question, and suggests that a significant percentage of people with schizophrenia will eventually have a substantial recovery. Manfred Bleuler (1968) reviewed pooled data from many studies and found that almost half of schizophrenic patients substantially improved or recovered. It has been suggested that the view that schizophrenia has a poor outcome is based on experience in public mental health clinics, which serve the 40 to 50 percent of people with schizophrenia who do poorly.

Etiology

Over the centuries, there have been a multitude of theories about the etiology of schizophrenia. These have ranged from religious, social, and psychological theories to more recent biological theories.

Early evidence of biological factors came from genetic studies. Twin studies showed that the rate of concordance was much higher for monozygotic (identical) than for dizygotic (fraternal) twins. Adoptive studies done by Kety et al. (1971) have shown that schizophrenia is much more prevalent in the biological relatives than in the adoptive families of those adopted at birth who are later diagnosed schizophrenic. Since that study, many others have shown biological differences between schizophrenic subjects and controls:

• CAT scans have demonstrated enlargement of the lateral ventricles and widened cortical sulci. This finding suggests either that there is brain atrophy or (more likely) that in some types of schizophrenia there has been abnormal brain development.

• PET scan studies have shown decreased activity in the frontal cortex.

• MRI scans have shown the presence of smaller anterior hippocampi (Weinberger et al. 1992) in schizophrenic subjects. Studies have also found a positive correlation between levels of HVA (a dopamine metabolite) in plasma and clinical severity.

The Dopamine Hypothesis

The dopamine hypothesis has been the predominant theory of biological causation for the past two decades. This theory hypothesizes that schizophrenia is caused by abnormal dopaminergic activity in the brain. Dopamine neurons are located in a number of different brain regions (see figure 3-E). In the basal ganglia, these nerve cells help to regulate motor functioning. In areas of the limbic and reticular systems, dopamine neurons appear to play an important role in emotional control and the screening of stimuli.

The dopamine theory holds that the basic physiological pathology involves primarily overactive or hyper-reactive dopamine neurons. The excessive dopamine activity can lead to behavioral agitation, a failure to adequately screen stimuli, and disorganization of perception and thought. This theory is supported by two observations: The first is that the potency of antipsychotic drugs has correlated closely with their ability to bind to and block the postsynaptic dopamine receptors in the mesolimbic system (see figure 9-A).

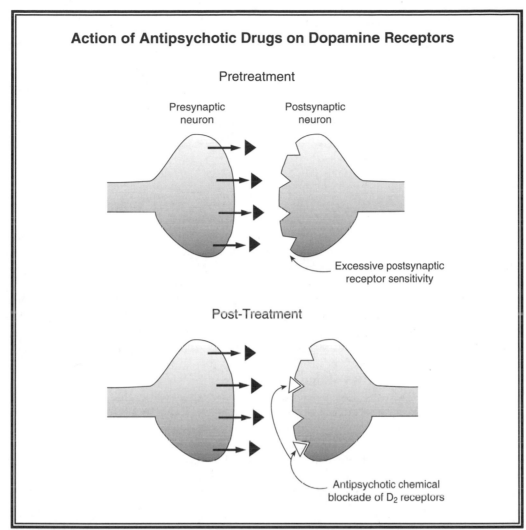

Action of Antipsychotic Drugs on Dopamine Receptors

Pretreatment

Presynaptic neuron

Postsynaptic neuron

Excessive postsynaptic receptor sensitivity

Post-Treatment

Antipsychotic chemical blockade of D_2 receptors

Figure 9-A

   The dopamine receptors in meso-limbic areas are referred to as D_2 receptors. The second observation is that drugs that increase dopamine activity (such as amphetamines) can product a paranoid psychosis similar to paranoid schizophrenia and, if given to schizophrenic patients, amphetamines may exacerbate psychotic symptoms.

   Although the dopamine theory has merit, the basic theory has recently been modified to help explain some clinical data (Davis et al. 1991). For many years it has been noted that a significant minority (about 30 percent) of schizophrenic patients do not respond well to standard antipsychotic medications. For the most part, these are patients who exhibit predominantly negative symptomatology. A number of researchers and clinicians assert that this group of patients may very well have a different type of underlying pathophysiology. In this group, the psychotic symptoms may be due to *hypo*dopaminergic activity in the prefrontal cortex, producing negative symptoms. The different neurochemical basis dictates alternative treatment approaches: the use of atypical antipsychotics (discussed in detail in chapter 17).

The Phencyclidine Theory

Another theory, proposed over 30 years ago (Luby et al. 1962), is the phencyclidine (PCP) model of schizophrenia. This is based on the discovery of a PCP receptor: the N-methyl-D-aspartate (NMDA) receptor, in the brain. Advantages of the PCP model are that, unlike amphetamines, PCP induces negativism and apathy in addition to disorganized thinking. It has been proposed (Javitt and Zukin 1991) that a primary NMDA dysregulation may lead to frontal cortex *hypo*dopaminergic activity and mesolimbic *hyper*dopaminergic activity. These questions remain to be clarified by future research.

Treatment

We can consider the positive and negative symptoms listed earlier as target symptoms for antipsychotic medication treatment. Antipsychotic medications are now considered an important, if not essential, component in the treatment of schizophrenia. The focus of treatment is not only the resolution of psychotic symptoms but also relapse prevention. Unfortunately, schizophrenia is a disorder in which relapse is extremely common. It is estimated that following a psychotic episode and subsequent recovery, 70 percent of patients will relapse within a year if treated with either placebo or no medication at all. With continued antipsychotic treatment the relapse rate can drop to 30 to 40 percent. Studies have shown that low-dose and intermittent treatment are associated with poorer outcome, as measured by number of hospitalizations (Carpenter et al. 1990; Kane 1990).

In addition, there is now evidence to support the notion that being psychotic is damaging to the brain (Loebel et al. 1992). It is as if the more the dopamine circuits are used, the more the psychotic pathways become etched into the brain. A. Loebel and associates studied the relationship between duration of illness and clinical outcome in a group of untreated, first-episode schizophrenic patients. The study showed that patients who had been psychotic longer prior to treatment tended to have a poorer treatment response. This is consistent with the observation that prolonged hallucinogen or stimulant abuse is associated with incomplete clearing of mental status. It also suggests some type of kindling phenomena or toxic effect of psychosis and supports the need for prompt treatment with antipsychotic medications.

Besides antipsychotic medications, both typical and atypical, other medications may be useful in the treatment of schizophrenia. These include lithium, carbamazepine, benzodiazepines, reserpine, propranolol, antidepressants, and antiparkinsonian drugs. Most of these are used to treat associated features of schizophrenia and are used in addition to, not instead of, antipsychotic medication. Lithium may be helpful to reduce psychotic and affective symptoms. It was once thought that lithium would benefit only those patients who were actually bipolar or schizoaffective, but even some patients without apparent affective symptoms can benefit from lithium. Benzopdiazepines (minor tranquilizers) may be helpful relieving some of the negative symptoms, in addition to anxiety and agitation. Antiparkinsonian medications are usually effective for the extrapyramidal side effects of antipsychotic medications. Antidepressants may be helpful when there are significant comorbid depressive symptoms. Propranolol (a beta blocker) is often helpful for akathisia (a common side effect of antipsychotic medications) and can sometimes reduce agitation.

The goal of medication treatment is to reduce symptoms so that the person can function better and benefit more from other forms of treatment, such as individual, group, or family therapy and social or vocational rehabilitation. An important part of such therapy involves educating the patient to prodromal symptoms and effects and side effects of medications. It is also important to address patients' beliefs that taking medications means they are sick (and conversely, that not taking medications means they aren't). Especially with paranoid patients, the belief that medications are a means of being controlled by others must be worked through.

Sometimes schizophrenics feel better not taking antipsychotic medications because they are able to entertain more grandiose notions about themselves and thereby lift their mood. Even more commonly, premature discontinuation occurs because patients are plagued by very unpleasant medication side effects. Like other people, they understandably don't like to suffer, and they respond by discontinuing. Appropriate education of patients regarding side effects and medical intervention (many side effects can be controlled with other medications) can improve the quality of life and greatly enhance compliance. It may be helpful to present medications as a tool for the person to use to help them control their illness, as a diabetic uses insulin.

Any of the psychotic disorders, regardless of etiology, may respond to antipsychotic medications. Where there is an underlying medical illness causing the psychosis, it is crucial to treat the underlying disorder. However, even in that case, antipsychotic medication may help reduce symptomatology. In the case of drug-induced and brief reactive psychosis, it may be appropriate not to use antipsychotic medications initially and instead to await the resolution of the psychotic symptoms using only supportive treatments. In the cases of the other psychoses, it is usually best to treat with antipsychotic medications for at least six months.

QUICK REFERENCE
When to Refer for Medication Treatment

Event	Symptoms
Organic psychosis	Delusions Hallucinations
Depression with psychotic features	Delusions Hallucinations Catatonic features
Schizophrenia	Positive symptoms
Other psychotic disorders	Delusions Hallucinations
Drug-induced state (including intoxication)	Severe paranoid delusions Hallucinations
Severe personality disorder	Disorganized thinking Prominent paranoia Poor impulse control
Manic episode	Prominent delusions Severe agitation

10

Post-Traumatic Stress Disorder

Natural disasters, catastrophic illnesses, incest, rape, and assault are but a few common life experiences that can unleash a wave of intense emotional stress. Acute stress reactions or "traumatic neuroses" were first addressed in the clinical literature during World War I, as thousands of soldiers returned from the front suffering from severe anxiety, insomnia, and nightmares attributed to "shell shock." The understanding of acute stress reactions was furthered by the pioneering work of Eric Lindeman.

In 1942, during an after-football celebration at the Coconut Grove nightclub in Boston, a disastrous fire claimed the lives of 499 people and stunned the community. Lindeman and his colleagues quickly rushed in and provided free counseling services for a large group of people, including survivors of the fire and relatives of the victims. At the same time they provided crisis intervention, the mental health team was able to carefully study this group of people. Lindeman discovered tremendous regularity in the symptoms that people reported: vacillation between overwhelming painful emotions and periods of numbness, a strong need or impulse to repeat the tragic events in their minds over and over again, nightmares, and a host of psychosomatic symptoms.

In 1976, psychiatrist Mardi Horowitz published a book entitled *Stress Response Syndromes*. In this landmark publication, Dr. Horowitz carved out a very useful model for understanding what appears to be a common pattern of human emotional response to significant stress and shed new light on the various aspects of PTSD symptomatology. Horowitz developed this model based on his review of numerous field studies (including Lindeman's), a good deal of clinical work treating mentally healthy people who had experienced major stresses, and even some experimental studies. Horowitz concluded that across a broad spectrum of stressful events (deaths of loved ones, physical assault, natural disaster, even viewing upsetting movies), most people exhibit a typical pattern of response. The various phases of the stress response syndrome helped to explain the differing and often dramatically shifting symptoms seen in PTSD.

Let's take a look at the stress response syndrome (see figure 10-A). The full stress response syndrome is seen most clearly in situations where the stressful event is sudden and intense. Although a host of events may trigger this reaction. Each of the boxes in the figure represents a state of mind or emotion. The stress response reaction begins with awareness of some painful event.

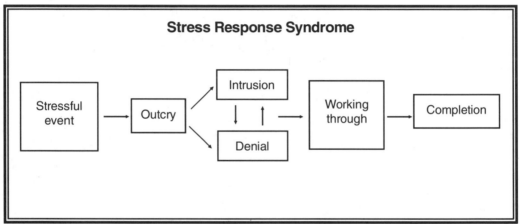

Figure 10-A

The first phase is Outcry. In a sense, a state of outcry is simultaneously an eruption of intense, unpleasant emotion (sadness, fear, and so on) *and* denial ("I can't believe it . . . it can't be true"). The person is in a state of shock and may be engulfed by very strong emotions. This phase of the reaction can last for a few minutes, a few hours, or a few days. Rather quickly, the person moves into phase two, which may be either a state of intrusion or a state of denial.

Intrusion occurs when a person experiences waves of intense emotion and a strong impulse to think about, imagine, remember, or mentally relive the stressful event. These experiences are deemed "intrusive" because generally the strong feelings and repetitive thoughts are not brought on willfully. During a state of intrusion, emotions feel very raw, and people feel extremely vulnerable, easily overwhelmed, and close to tears. They startle easily, don't sleep well, and often have nightmares. When intrusive experiences are especially intense, the individual may transiently lose reality testing and manifest psychotic-like symptoms, such as auditory or visual hallucinations.

Phase two includes a stage of Denial. Denial may occur directly following Outcry or may come on the heels of a period of intrusion. As noted earlier, denial is a state of emotional numbness; people often feel nothing. Other symptoms during the stages of denial include dissociative experiences (feelings of detachment, estrangement, impaired concentration, forgetfulness), avoidance of situations that may be associated with the trauma, and marked general social withdrawal.

Although *DSM-IV* includes post-traumatic stress disorder as an anxiety disorder, in some respects this may be a misnomer. Clearly, anxiety symptoms predominate in PTSD, but it is very common for PTSD patients to exhibit major depression, transient psychosis, and substance abuse as well. The symptoms of PTSD can be organized into six categories, as follows:

Symptoms of PTSD

- Persistent reexperiencing of the trauma
  - Distressing, intrusive recollections of the event (images, affects, cognitions)
  - Recurring nightmares regarding the trauma
  - "Flashbacks" or déjà vu (sensations as if the traumatic episode were happening in the present)

- Increased arousal
  - Sleep disturbances
  - Startle response
  - Irritability
  - Hypervigilance

- Transient psychotic symptoms
  - Derealization
  - Illusions
  - Hallucinations (visual or auditory)

- Avoidance
  - Avoiding discussion of the traumatic events
  - Avoiding activities or people and places that could provoke recollections of the trauma
  - General social withdrawal

- Numbing
  - Blunted affective responses
  - Feelings of emptiness
  - Feelings of estrangement or detachment
  - Clouding of consciousness

- Associated features
  - Major depression
  - Panic attacks
  - Substance abuse (often seen as an attempt to "self-medicate," to reduce anxiety or intrusive experiences)

Differential Diagnosis

PTSD is subdivided into the following clinical presentations: acute (duration of symptoms is less than three
months) and chronic (duration of symptoms is more
than three months). Also two versions of PTSD are
seen clinically: acute onset (the traumatic event has
just recently occurred) and delayed onset (the onset
of severe symptoms occurs at least six months after
the traumatic event). Beyond these distinctions, other
variables are extremely important to consider both in
terms of diagnosis and treatment.

Lenore Terr (1991) aptly notes that *generally* sin-
gle-blow traumas have a less devastating effect on
psychologic functioning than recurring traumas. In
the latter case are situations such as repeated child
abuse and molestation, systematic terrorizing, and recurring spousal abuse. The age at which trauma occurs also plays a crucial role in our understanding of
psychological sequelae. Very early, severe, recurring
child abuse often not only results in primary symptoms of PTSD but may also interfere significantly with
fundamental personality development. The outcome
may be coexisting PTSD and borderline or other severe personality disorder.

Since PTSD can have a variety of symptomatic
presentations (owing to the above-mentioned variables and whether the person is in the intrusion or
denial stage of the stress response syndrome), it is
wise first to formulate the overall diagnosis and then
delineate particular target symptoms (see symptom
list, above). In all forms of PTSD, ultimately the psychiatric symptoms can be traced to the patient's exposure to extremely overwhelming psychosocial
stressors. And in almost all cases, a common element
is the person's experience of extraordinary helplessness or powerlessness in the face of such stressors.

Etiology

Volumes have been written about the psychological
origins and consequences of severe trauma, and it is
beyond the scope of this book to attempt a review.
Suffice it to say that the majority of PTSD symptoms
can be understood as arising largely from psychogenic
sources. However, some authors have proposed inter-
esting theories regarding biological factors in PTSD, which we will review here. The
primary work in this area has been done by Bessel A. van der Kolk (1987). In this
chapter we will look at five models in which biology potentially can be altered by
psychological stress.

Attachment and the repetition compulsion

PTSD due to early, severe child abuse or neglect may leave not only emotional scars; neurobiology may be altered. Severe stress during childhood and infancy in both humans and animals can result in an increased need for attachment and protection. Studies with birds, dogs, and monkeys show that infants will strongly seek out attachments even with abusive parents, especially under stress. "Thus attachment remains strong, even when the imprinted object no longer provides effective protection and nurturance" (van der Kolk 1987). This behavioral pattern seen so strongly in other species, may provide some understanding of the common human tendency for abused individuals to cling to and gravitate toward abusive parents and spouses. Since it is seen across diverse species, this may reflect an underlying neurobiologically mediated reaction pattern.

The repetitive involvement in apparently aversive or abusive relationships (sometimes called the repetition compulsion) may be related to hypersensitivity of the separation-stress center in the brain (see the discussion in chapter 7), which has been shown to respond favorably to treatment with antidepressants, especially MAO inhibitors.

Attachment and impaired affect modulation

When the traumatic experience has occurred early in life, another consequence, conversely, may be inadequate attachment and bonding. This may be especially true if the nature of the trauma was profound neglect. One common consequence of inadequate or insecure attachment is poor affective regulation. Studies with monkeys have revealed that isolated, neglected infants often develop persistent aggressive and self-destructive behaviors (such as biting) and, in general, impaired abilities for emotional regulation. Clearly many PTSD patients also show chronic problems with emotional control and at times manifest symptoms of self-mutilation (Harlow and Harlow 1971; Sackett 1965). This may account for both chronic emotional arousal and an increased vulnerability to later traumatic life events (van der Kolk 1987).

Hyperarousal

When animals are exposed to inescapable shock, they exhibit consistent behavioral reactions—initially hypervigilance or arousal and ultimately a profound state of withdrawal and "depression." In addition, such animals eventually show a significant depletion of norepinephrine, likely accompanied by changes in NE receptor sensitivity in parts of the brain. Alterations of receptor sensitivity may leave the animals in a state of chronic hyperarousal. In essence, their nervous systems may be permanently altered such that traumatized animals and people alike are relatively unable to dampen or inhibit excessive emotional arousal. Antidepressants that affect norepinephrine appear to alter receptor sensitivity, both in humans and animals. Serotonergic antidepressants may also indirectly inhibit hypersensitive NE cells (Nagy et al. 1993), and thus can play a role in treating hyperarousal in PTSD patients.

Intrusive symptoms

L. M. Nagy et al. (1993) report that PTSD patients treated with high doses of fluoxetine (a serotonergic antidepressant) showed a significant reduction in flashbacks and other intrusive symptoms. Interestingly, as intrusive experiences decreased so did symptoms of avoidance and numbing. (Again, the reductions were at levels that were statistically significant.) Furthermore, van der Kolk (1987) has hypothesized that flashback experiences may be traced (neurobiologically) to "stress-induced reaction of LC—hippocampus/amygdala pathways." As we saw in chapter 7, the locus coeruleus is mediated by norepinephrine, and selective serotonin antidepressants also clearly have an inhibitory effect on LC activation.

Kindling

Finally, it has been hypothesized that severely traumatic experiences may result in a sort of kindling effect, in which repeated episodes of trauma literally change brain functioning and even brain morphology. Severe trauma may *progressively* increase the likelihood that subsequent stresses are responded to with even more intense affective symptoms (see chapter 2). Animal models have suggested a kindling effect following emotional trauma (for instance, Kraemer et al. 1984), although at present this theory remains mostly speculative. There are clinical and anecdotal reports that some PTSD patients benefit from treatment with lithium carbonate, clonazepam, and carbamazepine, all of which have been shown to inhibit kindling effects.

Summary

Animal models strongly support the notion that severely traumatic experiences alter brain functioning and may more or less permanently change an organism's biologic capacity for response to stressful stimuli. It is likely that this occurs for human beings as well, although definitive conclusions await more sophisticated human studies. Thus, although PTSD can be seen as *induced by* environmental-psychologic stressors, the *impact* is on both psyche and soma. The resulting disorder is best understood as a psychological and neurobiological problem.

Treatment

The treatment of choice for PTSD is psychotherapy. It is essential that these patients gradually come to face the painful memories of traumatic experiences—come to terms with the realities of their lives. The process of "working through" is often quite prolonged and fraught with periodic emotional upheaval. Typically PTSD pa-

---

PTSD Symptoms That Respond to Medication

Target Symptoms	Class of Medication
Intrusive experiences "flashbacks"[a] and avoidance and numbing[b]	5-HT antidepressants
Hyperarousal[c]	Antidepressants, benzodiazepines such as clonazepam
Transient psychosis, marked derealization	Low dose antipsychotics
Depression[d]	Antidepressants
Panic Attacks	Antidepressants, MAO inhibitors, high-potency benzodiazepines

[a] Nagy et al. (1993); Davidson et al. (1991)
[b] As intrusive symptoms are reduced and affective control improves, often numbing and avoidance diminish.
[c] van der Kolk (1987)
[d] Davidson et al. (1990)

Figure 10-B

tients must navigate through repeated periods of intrusion and denial on their way toward psychological resolution and symptomatic improvement. During this treatment, it is crucial that affective reexperiencing of painful events be "dosed" (gradual, paced exposure) so as to not overwhelm or retraumatize the patient. Medications can be used in treating certain aspects of PTSD, but are not the primary treatment. In all cases, psychotropic medications should target particular, serious symptoms *as they arise*. Figure 10-B summarizes common target symptoms and provides treatment implications drawn from the very limited studies and clinical experience available.

Central to appropriate pharmacological treatment of PTSD is the restoration of some sense of control over turbulent emotions. When medications are appropriately used, in the context of a solid and safe patient-therapist relationship, the improved emotional control can serve as a sort of antidote for what is otherwise a feeling of powerlessness. Ultimately, the ability to face painful realities with a degree of mastery is at the heart of recovery from PTSD.

At times, excessively high doses of benzodiazepines or antipsychotics have been used (often inappropriately) in desperate attempts to snuff out eruptions of painful affect. This approach can backfire, as it results in a chemically induced state of "dissociation." The patient may then be unable to access inner emotions or memories, and the process of working through comes to a halt. Also, overly aggressive medication treatment can be experienced by the patient as an assault in its own right—another case of being controlled by a powerful other. In cases of extremely severe intrusive symptoms or psychosis, aggressive pharmacotherapy may be necessary, but it should be seen only as a short-term solution that continues only until the patient has regained a measure of stability. At that time the dosage of benzodiazepines or antipsychotics should be reduced.

When the PTSD patient develops a full-blown clinical depression or a severe, entrenched panic disorder, antidepressants can be quite helpful. When PTSD patients are treated with antidepressants, the course of treatment almost invariably must be lengthy (as in treating all panic disorders and major depression)—at least nine to twelve months (see chapters 5 and 14).

QUICK REFERENCE
When to Refer for Medication Treatment

Psychotherapy is the treatment of choice for most cases of PTSD. Psychotropic medications can be used when the patient presents with any of the following:

- Persistent ego weakness and an inability to tolerate exploratory psychotherapy.

- Low level of cognitive functioning and an inability to benefit from exploratory psychotherapy.

- When the following target symptoms become too intense and overwhelming or markedly interfere with functioning in daily life, *short-term* medication treatment is indicated:

  Intrusive experiences, flashbacks
  Transient psychosis
  Marked derealization
  Avoidance and numbing

- When these target symptoms become too intense and overwhelming or markedly interfere with functioning in daily life, *longer-term* medication treatment is indicated:

  Major depression
  Panic disorder
  Persistent psychotic symptoms

11

Borderline Personality Disorders

The concept of borderline disorders has slowly emerged from Hoch's early description of pseudoneurotic schizophrenia and Grinker's landmark study in 1968. Nosological and theoretical controversy has surrounded this very common diagnostic group. It has often been referred to as a "wastebasket" diagnosis—a depository for those clients who are severely impaired, hard to diagnose, or especially difficult to treat. All therapists encounter people with severe levels of character pathology. These folks are said to exhibit a very "loud" form of psychopathology; they suffer a lot and cause great suffering in others. According to Allan Francis (1989) borderline patients often seek out psychotherapy and psychotropic medication treatment—and often overdose on both!

Differential Diagnosis

Borderline disorders have been viewed both from a behavioral-symptomatic perspective (such as that of *DSM-IV*) and a theoretical perspective (for example, borderline personality organization à la Kernberg and others). As Grinker and many subsequent researchers and clinicians agree, borderline patients are not all alike; they present in many different sizes and shapes. You can see borderline characteristics in the context of a number of different personality styles: schizoid-detached, obsessional, paranoid, narcissistic, and histrionic. However, all varieties share a few common characteristics:

Borderline Personality Disorders Facts

- The incidence of severe personality disorders in the general population is difficult to determine. However, in some community mental health clinics, up to 25 percent of clients present with an Axis II borderline personality disorder.

- Among borderline patients, the lifetime mortality rate by suicide is between 10 and 15 percent.

- Recent longitudinal studies suggest that two-thirds of borderline patients experience a significant reduction in emotional instability and impulsivity after age 45. Thus appropriate crisis management and supportive medication treatment can play an important role in sustaining functioning and survival until patients reach their fourth decade.

Core Symptoms of Borderline Personality Disorders

- Generalized ego impairment
- Chronic emotional instability
- Chaotic interpersonal relations
- Feelings of emptiness
- Impaired sense of self
- Low frustration tolerance
- Impulsivity
- Primitive defenses, such as splitting, acting out
- Irritability and anger-control problems

Beyond these commonalties are a considerable variety of symptomatic presentations. The particular behaviors observed are colored by the patient's style (obsessional, histrionic, and so on), the nature of their current social support network, and the presence or absence of comorbid Axis I disorders.

The critical defining feature that can help the clinician be more certain of a borderline diagnosis is the history. As noted in chapter 4, many individuals may transiently experience borderline characteristics while in the throes of a major Axis I disorder (for example, a depression), only to recompensate when the Axis I problem resolves. A more definitive diagnosis of borderline disorder emerges when there is a well-documented history of ego impairment dating back to adolescence or early adulthood—"stable instability."

DSM-IV presents but one version of borderline disorder (a type of histrionic-dependent borderline). Speaking more broadly in this book, we will refer to borderline disorders as including a host of personality "styles" that share the common core features listed above. In addition, it is helpful to delineate three subgroups of borderlines. These subgroups have been derived both by research methods (cluster and factor analysis) and by a method that psychopharmacologist Donald Klein calls "pharmacological behavioral dissection." This latter approach looks at how different groups of patients respond to psychotropic medications; based on their response patterns, subtypes can be identified.

Hysteroid-dysphoric

These borderline clients present with a significant degree of emotional lability and are exquisitely sensitive to interpersonal rejection, loss, and abandonment. As a consequence, they often cannot tolerate being alone and may engage in desperate attempts to maintain attachments, including clinging behavior and manipulative suicidal threats or gestures. These patients are at great risk for recurring depression.

Schizotypal

These borderline patients chronically display odd thinking—ideas of reference, magical thinking, vagueness, very idiosyncratic beliefs—and periodically experience marked episodes of depersonalization or derealization and transient psychoses. Such people likely represent a truer sort of borderline schizophrenia.

Angry-impulsive

These people are characterized by their pervasively hostile-aggressive way of interacting with others. They have very low frustration tolerance and can be quite volatile. As a result, their interpersonal relations are replete either with ongoing intense friction or multiple rejections.

In addition to these subtypes, it is important to keep in mind that many, if not most, borderline personalities have comorbid Axis I disorders—especially common are major depression and substance abuse. These coexisting disorders always complicate the picture and must be dealt with in any approach to treatment. In particular, longitudinal studies following the course and outcome of borderline personality disorders over the life span suggest very clearly that those patients who continue to do poorly are those who continue to abuse alcohol and other substances. Thus treatment of chemical dependency problems *must* be addressed.

Etiology

Most writings addressing the etiology of borderline disorders focus on psychological factors—especially traumatic events and serious developmental failures in the early family of origin (Mahler, Kernberg, Kohut, Masterson, and so on). Biological theories are, at this time, only speculative. They include the following:

- In-born or constitutional factors in the CNS may leave certain children with defects in their ability to psychologically "metabolize" early interpersonal experiences adequately. Thus, even if raised in a "good enough" home, some kids simply may not acquire adequate emotional nurturance and sustainment from otherwise good parents.

- In-born or constitutional factors may lead to the development of a difficult temperamental style, such as an irritable, restless infant. Some children cry excessively, seem extremely sensitive to mild stressors, or are unable to be soothed. There certainly are times when such children evoke ongoing negative reactions in otherwise good parents: (frustration, withdrawal of affection, and so on). Thus the child is both biologically at risk (less capable of handling stress, more sensitive) and prone toward behaving in ways that may provoke less-than-optimal parental interactions or bonding. The secondary parental-child friction likely contributes to ongoing problems with psychological growth.

- Early, severely traumatic experiences *may* literally alter brain development, resulting in chronic neurotransmitter abnormalities (Stone 1988; see chapter 10).

In the theories above, the particular biological-based abnormalities or dysfunctions may become manifest in various symptom clusters, as noted earlier: hysteroid-dysphoria, schizotypal, and angry-impulsive. It may be hypothesized that these subtypes of borderline disorders have neurochemical abnormalities, as outlined in figure 11-A. It must be emphasized, however, that at present such theories are quite speculative and not yet verified by well-controlled studies. Many studies attempting to identify biological markers in borderline disorders have shown inconclusive results. These results are largely due to designs in which diagnostic subtypes are col-

---

Hypothesized Neurochemical Dysfunctions of Borderline Disorder Subtypes

Subtype	Neurotransmitter	Location
Hysteroid-dysphoria	NE	Locus coeruleus
Schizotypal	DA	Mesolimbic and reticular formation
Angry-impulsive	5-HT	Amygdala

Figure 11-A

lapsed into an overly heterogeneous group of patients in which there is no control for comorbid Axis I disorders.

Treatment

No medication treatment can directly treat personality disorders, per se. Rather, psychotropic medications are used to ameliorate certain target symptoms. From results of the limited studies available, the medications of choice appear to be those listed in the Quick Reference. The reduction in target symptoms can contribute significantly to improved coping ability and reduced levels of emotional despair. It is clear that no magic pill can cure deep characterological wounds, but targeted medication treatment of borderline patients can be an important adjunct to psychotherapy and crisis management.

Cautions

Three cautions are important to note:

- Treatment with antianxiety medications (benzodiazepines) is risky with borderline patients. These patients are certainly at risk for tranquilizer abuse. In addition, clinical experience, as well as research, shows that benzodiazepines can contribute to emotional dyscontrol and increased suicidality with borderline patients (Cowdry and Gardner 1988).

- Since many borderline patients are at risk for transient psychosis, the antidepressant bupropion (a dopamine agonist) should be used with caution. This drug, which is an effective antidepressant, may precipitate psychosis in prepsychotic individuals.

- Because this group as a whole engages in frequent suicidal acting out, it is advisable to treat borderline patients with medications that have been found to have a low degree of toxicity when taken in overdose. These include antipsychotics and the following antidepressants: fluoxetine, paroxetine, bupropion (note above caution), trazodone, and sertraline. Most other antidepressants are quite toxic when taken in overdose.

QUICK REFERENCE
Medications for Treating Borderline Subtypes

Borderline Subtype	Class of Medication
Hysteroid-dysphoria[a]	MAO inhibitors, carbamazepine (anticonvulsant)
Schizotypal[b]	Low doses of antipsychotics
Angry-impulsive[c]	5-HT antidepressants
Comorbid major depression	Antidepressants
Comorbid panic disorder	Antidepressants

[a] Cowdry and Gardner 1988; Gardner and Cowdry 1986; Liebowitz and Klein 1981
[b] Soloff et al. 1986; Francis and Soloff 1988; Goldberg et al. 1986
[c] Norden 1989; Cornelius et al. 1991

12

Substance-Related Disorders

Substance abuse and related disorders represent a major problem area facing the clinician. Despite the "war on drugs" they continue to be a widespread problem: At least 5 percent of Americans are alcoholic, and stimulant abuse is a serious problem among teenagers and young adults. Any solution to these problems will undoubtedly involve social and political factors in addition to clinical programs. This chapter focuses on the differing types of clinical syndromes related to each commonly abused substance and medications that may be useful as an adjunct to treatment.

Often the clinician will be confronted with a client who has substance-use problems in addition to the psychiatric disorder (comorbidity or dual diagnosis) or whose psychiatric disorder may be a direct result of substance use. In either case, treatment of the substance disorder will be crucial to the treatment of the psychiatric disorder. In the past, substance use was often seen as a form of self-medication—the person was using the drug to "treat" an emotional disorder, and psychotherapy was attempted in an effort to cure the person of the need for the substance—usually to no avail. In recent years, the evidence has shown that achieving abstinence is frequently a precondition for effectively dealing with psychological issues. In fact, the emotional problems may be significantly diminished by the person's achieving abstinence. For example, most (but not all) alcohol-related depression resolves within one to two weeks of abstinence. The interaction between substance-related disorders and other psychiatric disorders (like that between Axis I and Axis II disorders) is a complex one. We try here to clarify some of the more well-defined relationships.

Substance-Abuse Facts

- Alcoholism affects 5 to 10 percent of the adult population.

- Alcoholism plays a major role in the following causes of death: accidents, homicide, suicide, and alcoholic cirrhosis.

- One million Americans are reported to be addicted to cocaine, and over five million use cocaine regularly.

- Billions of dollars are spent annually on the treatment and prosecution of drug users.

- 30 to 50 percent of those in mental health treatment have a significant substance-abuse disorder.

Differential Diagnosis

Substance-related disorders are divided in *DSM-IV* into dependence, abuse, intoxication, and withdrawal. In addition, each substance may have related disorders phenomenologically similar to other disorders: delirium, dementia, amnestic, psychotic, mood, anxiety, sex, and sleep disorders.

Substance dependence is defined in *DSM-IV* as a pattern of substance use leading to significant impairment or distress, demonstrated by at least three of the following:

- Tolerance—diminished effect from the same amount of the substance, often leading to use of increased amounts to achieve the same effect

- Withdrawal—onset of withdrawal syndrome if the substance is discontinued, often leading to continued use to avoid withdrawal symptoms

- Substance is taken more than intended

- Persistent use despite efforts to cut down

- Great deal of effort is expended to obtain or continue use of the substance, or recover from its effects

- Other important activities are reduced in order to continue substance use

- Continued substance use despite knowledge that it is harmful

The *DSM-IV* defines *substance abuse* as a pattern of substance use leading to significant impairment or distress, demonstrated by at least one of the following:

- Impairment of home, work, or school performance as a result of substance use

- Hazardous behavior resulting from substance use

- Legal problems resulting from substance use

- Continued substance use despite significant resultant problems

Intoxication refers to an acutely altered mental state due to ingestion of (or exposure to) a substance that is not caused by a medical condition or other mental disorder.

Withdrawal refers to an altered state produced by cessation or reduction of use of a substance which causes significant impairment in functioning in important areas and is not caused by a medical condition or other mental disorder. The disorder may be "persisting"—may continue even though substance use has stopped and the withdrawal syndrome has been resolved.

Figures 12-A and 12-B list substances and the clinical syndromes they can produce. Not all substances can cause every syndrome. For example, phencyclidine (PCP) can produce a very severe psychosis during intoxication but has no withdrawal syn-

Major Substance Diagnoses

Substance	Dependence	Abuse	Intoxication	Withdrawal	Persisting
Alcohol	X	X	X	X	X
Hallucinogens	X	X	X		X
Opioids	X	X	X	X	
Phencyclidine	X	X	X		
Sedative-hypnotics	X	X	X	X	X
Stimulants	X	X	X	X	

Figure 12-A

Substance-Induced Disorders That Mimic Other Disorders

Substance	Delirium	Dementia	Amnestic	Psychotic	Mood	Anxiety
Alcohol	X	X	X	X	X	X
Hallucinogens	X			X	X	X
Opioids	X			X	X	
Phencyclidine	X			X	X	X
Sedative-hypnotics	X	X	X	X	X	X
Stimulants	X			X	X	X

Figure 12-B

drome; whereas sedative-hypnotics (such as benzodiapines) can produce all of the substance diagnoses, as can alcohol. In the remainder of this chapter we review several of the major classes of substances associated with clinical disorders.

Alcohol

Alcohol (ethanol) is a water-soluble substance that is rapidly absorbed and readily crosses the blood-brain barrier. It is a CNS depressant and is metabolized by the liver. It is also a gastric irritant and is toxic to liver cells and neurons. Alcohol is probably the most-studied substance of abuse (and the most abused substance). It is associated with dependence, abuse, withdrawal, intoxication, delirium, dementia, amnesia, delusions, hallucinations, mood disorder, anxiety disorder, sexual dysfunction, and sleep disorder.

There is much evidence demonstrating that alcoholism is familial, but the exact biological mechanism remains unclear. Several studies have tried to find a biological marker for alcoholism. Studies have shown a differential sensitivity to alcohol in alcoholics versus nonalcoholics (Pollock 1992). M. A. Schuckit, E. Gold, and C. Risch (1987) have shown that sons of alcoholics had significantly lower prolactin levels in response to ethanol challenge. Smith et al. (1992) showed that alcoholics were more likely to show *Taq* 1 A1 restriction fragment length polymorphism of the D_2 dopamine receptor gene (and dopamine controls prolactin release). The significance of these findings, however, remains speculative, and the search continues for the biological basis of alcoholism.

Psychiatric symptoms are very common in alcohol intoxication and withdrawal, but studies by Schuckit show that most of these symptoms improve greatly within one to four weeks of abstinence and are likely to abate over several months (Brown and Schuckit 1988; Schuckit, Irwin, and Brown 1990). The three diagnoses associated with increased risk of alcoholism are schizophrenia, mania, and antisocial personality disorder. As a depressant, alcohol tends to produce depressive symptoms during intoxication and anxiety symptoms during withdrawal and abstinence. These syndromes often mimic major depression or an anxiety disorder, but they will usually resolve within two weeks of abstinence and do not require prolonged treatment.

Medications can play an important role in the treatment of alcohol-related disorders. Figure 12-C lists medications that can be used in the treatment of alcohol-related disorders. Most of those medications are covered in part three of this book. The exception is disulfiram (Antabuse), a medication used to assist in the maintenance of abstinence. Disulfiram causes an accumulation of acetaldehyde if a person drinks alcohol while taking it, which leads to an unpleasant and potentially dangerous reaction involving flushing, throbbing headache, nausea, and vomiting. Only certain people are appropriate for disulfiram treatment. Some are able to remain

---

Alcohol-Related Disorders and Medications for Treating Them

Disorder	Medication
Intoxication	Thiamine, folate, multivitamins
Withdrawal	Benzodiazepines
Abstinence maintenance	Antabuse, naltrexone,[a] lithium,[a] SSRIs[a]
Delirium	Benzodiazepines
Dementia	—
Amnesia	Thiamine
Delusional disorder	Benzodiazepines, antipsychotics
Hallucinosis	Benzodiazepines, antipsychotics
Mood disorder	Antidepressants[a]
Anxiety disorder	Benzodiazepines, buspirone

[a] Likely, but not proven

Figure 12-C

abstinent without it; some will drink in spite of it. In between are those who will be able to reinforce their desire for abstinence by taking disulfiram 250 to 500 mg once daily. Naltrexone, an opiate antagonist, has also shown some promise in helping maintain abstinence by reducing craving for alcohol (Bender 1993).

Stimulants

Amphetamines ("crank," "speed," "bennies") and cocaine ("crack," "freebase") have become common substances of abuse. They are CNS stimulants that act on the dopaminergic system. Research suggests that a dopamine-medicated endogenous reward system in the limbic system is activated by amphetamines and cocaine. Amphetamines produce increased release of dopamine and norepinephrine along with their attendant peptides, and decreased re-uptake. This leads to increased dopaminergic and noradrenergic activity and symptoms of euphoria, paranoia, and hyperexcitability. The half-life of dextroamphetamine is about ten hours. Cocaine produces similar pharmacologic effects but has a shorter duration of action and in some forms, especially crack cocaine, produces more intense effects thus making it more addictive.

To understand the pharmacologic treatment of stimulant dependency it is helpful to look at the different phases of use on a neuronal level (see figure 12-D). During acute intoxication there is increased release of catecholamines (dopamine and norepinephrine) and enkephalins, along with decreased re-uptake, leading to increased catecholamine activity. In the acute withdrawal state there is a reduction of available neurotransmitters (due to depletion and reduced reuptake). This leaves a state of reduced catecholamine activity and feelings of craving, depression, and restlessness. With chronic use, there is development of tolerance, further reduced availability of neurotransmitter, and an increased number of receptors (supersensitivity) leading to lower occupancy and feelings of craving, depression, and anhedonia.

Pharmacological treatment of stimulant use is different for each phase of use. During acute intoxication, medications can be used to block the effects of dopamine and norepinephrine. During withdrawal, medications are used to reduce craving (and hopefully subsequent use). The medications used to treat amphetamine use (see figure 12-E) generally potentiate the effects of norepinephrine, dopamine, or both. Most

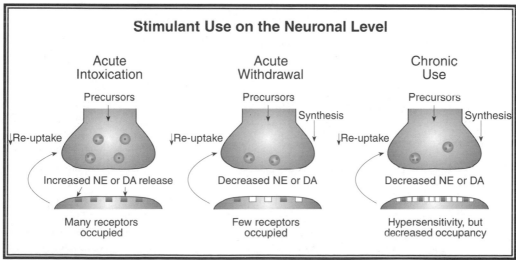

Stimulant Use on the Neuronal Level

Acute Intoxication	Acute Withdrawal	Chronic Use
Precursors	Precursors	Precursors
	Synthesis	Synthesis
↓Re-uptake	↓Re-uptake	↓Re-uptake
Increased NE or DA release	Decreased NE or DA	Decreased NE or DA
Many receptors occupied	Few receptors occupied	Hypersensitivity, but decreased occupancy

Figure 12-D

Medications Used to Treat Phases of Stimulant Use

State	Medications
Intoxication	Beta blockers
	Clonidine
	Benzodiazepines
	Antipsychotics
Withdrawal	Desipramine
	Other antidepressants
	Bromocriptine
	Amantadine
	Lithium
	L-dopa
	Carbamazepine

Figure 12-E

of those medications are discussed in part three of this book. Bromocriptine is a D_2 dopamine agonist. Amantadine increases dopamine activity. L-dopa is a dopamine precursor that leads to increased dopamine synthesis. All these medications increase dopamine activity, thereby reducing the feelings of craving produced by dopamine depletion. It should be noted, however, that dopaminergic medications can produce psychotic symptoms, so the dose must be monitored closely. The effectiveness of these medications continues to be under investigation. They are not a panacea, but are often helpful in reducing symptoms of withdrawal and craving.

Opiates

Heroin was first synthesized from morphine over a century ago. Since then, it has become one of the most abused substances. Research into why it produces such powerful effects has lead to the discovery of specific opiate receptors and endogenous opioids (enkephalins and endorphins). These peptides appear to be neurotransmitters involved with the sensation of pain and pleasure. A number of opiates and synthetic opioids are available and can lead to dependency, including morphine, heroin, propoxyphene (Darvon), methadone, meperidine (Demerol), pentazocine (Talwin), hydromorphone (Dilaudid), oxycodone (Percodan), and hydrocodone (Vicodin, Damason-P), and codeine.

Different medications are used to treat different phases of opiate use (see figure 12-F). Acute opiate (opioid) intoxication leads to sedation, pupillary constriction, and respiratory depression and can be fatal. There are specific opiate antagonists that block the opiate receptors and rapidly reverse these effects: naloxone and naltrexone. Opiate withdrawal is characterized by anxiety, agitation, sweating, gastrointestinal upset, tremulousness, running nose. It is treated by using an opiate such as propoxyphene (Darvon), methadone, or clonidine, or a combination of these drugs.

There are two strategies for treating dependence or abuse. One is to use methadone, a long-acting synthetic opiate that is well tolerated and reduces craving for other opiates such as heroin. Methadone is used for maintenance treatment because, with its long half-life, it produces less of a "high" and is less prone to abuse. It is

```
+-------------------------------------------------------------------------+
|            Medications Used to Treat Phases of Opiate Use                |
|   State                          Medication                             |
|                                                                         |
|   Acute intoxication             Naloxone (injectable)                  |
|                                  Naltrexone (oral)                      |
|   Acute withdrawal               Opiates, especially methadone and      |
|                                  propoxyphene                           |
|                                  Clonidine                              |
|                                  Benzodiazepines                        |
|   Maintaining abstinence         Methadone                              |
|                                  Naloxone or naltrexone                 |
+-------------------------------------------------------------------------+
```

Figure 12-F

now available only in certain federally approved treatment sites. The other is to have the client take an opiate antagonist (naloxone or naltrexone) so that the effect of the opiate will be blocked if it is used.

Hallucinogens

Various substances can produce transient psychotic states, often accompanied by visual, auditory, or olfactory hallucinations. These include LSD (lysergic acid diethylamide), mescaline, psilocybin, and PCP. These drugs are not associated with dependence or withdrawal, but they can produce a florid psychosis during acute intoxication. This effect can usually be allowed to run its course (usually twelve to twenty-four hours), but sometimes medications (such as antianxiety or antipsychotic) need to be used to decrease agitation and stabilize blood pressure.

Sometimes patients will report a reexperiencing or "flashback" of hallucinations they had during a previous ingestion of hallucinogen. These reactions likewise usually do not require treatment with medication but, when severe, may benefit from antianxiety or antipsychotic medication. Severe overdoses of PCP can lead to convulsions and may require emergency medical treatment.

Other Drugs

Other substances of abuse—including caffeine, cannabis, inhalants, and nicotine—are not covered here since they are less important clinically. Caffeine intoxication can lead to anxiety or confusion. Inhalants can cause an organic psychosis and are very neurotoxic—leading to permanent neurological deficit. Nicotine dependence can be treated with a nicotine gum or patch (in conjunction with cognitive-behavioral treatment). Sedative abuse and dependence is discussed in chapter 16, on antianxiety medications.

QUICK REFERENCE
Treatment of Substance-Related Disorders

	Symptoms	Treatment
Alcohol		
Intoxication	Confusion, slurred speech, ataxia, delirium	Supportive thiamine, vitamins
Withdrawal	Anxiety, agitation, possible hallucinations, possible convulsions	Benzodiazepines
Stimulants		
Intoxication	Anxiety, agitation	Supportive; benzodiazepines, beta blockers, clonidine
	Paranoid psychosis	Antipsychotics
Withdrawal	Anergia, irritabililty	Supportive amantadine, bromocriptine
	Depressed mood	Cyclic antidepressants
Opiates		
Intoxication	Sedation, respiratory depression	Naloxone, naltrexone
Withdrawal	Anxiety, agitation, sweating, tremors	Clonidine, benzodiazepines, opiates (methadone or propoxyphene)
Hallucinogens		
Intoxication	Agitation, prominent hallucinations	Benzodiazepines, antipsychotics
Withdrawal	No withdrawal syndrome	

13

Other Miscellaneous Disorders

There are several types of disorders that, although they are encountered less often in clinical practice, we have chosen to discuss in this chapter. Compared to disorders discussed in earlier chapters, their biological basis is less well understood at this time, and the role of medications may be less clear. These disorders are: Tourette's syndrome, eating disorders (anorexia and bulimia nervosa), attention deficit disorder (ADD), and self-mutilation.

Tourette's Syndrome

Tourette's (or Gilles de la Tourette) syndrome is characterized by motor and vocal tics—sudden involuntary movements or vocalizations. It is most known for coprolalia (sudden yelling of obscenities), but this is only seen in 25 to 30 percent of cases. Motor tics typically involve the head and neck. Vocal tics may be guttural sounds, repeated coughing, or words. Tourette's is now generally considered a neurological disorder, although symptoms may be exacerbated by anxiety or tension. It appears to involve dysfunction of dopaminergic pathways and is treated with dopamine D_2 blockers—haloperidol or pimozide, in low to moderate doses. Persons with Tourette's have a higher incidence of obsessive-compulsive disorder—a finding not well understood at this time.

Eating Disorders

Eating disorders are divided into two main types in *DSM-IV:* anorexia nervosa and bulimia nervosa. Anorexia nervosa involves significant weight loss and maintenance of a very low body weight, by restriction of intake, purging, or both, often in combination with excessive exercising.

The *DSM-IV* diagnostic criteria are:

- Body weight less than 85 percent of that expected

- Fear of gaining weight

- Distorted perception of one's weight (thinking one is fat when actually very thin)

- Missing at least three consecutive menstrual cycles (where applicable)

Bulimia nervosa involves repeated episodes of binging and purging: eating large amounts of food (everything in the refrigerator) and then purging through self-induced vomiting or use of laxatives or diuretics. In addition (*DSM-IV*):

- Both the binge eating and compensatory behaviors occur, on average, at least twice a week for three months.

- Self-esteem is overly influenced by weight.

- Disturbance does not occur only during periods of anorexia nervosa.

Much research has investigated personality characteristics, psychological issues, family dynamics, and the biological basis of anorexia and bulimia. Anorexia usually requires a multimodal, if not a multidisciplinary, treatment approach. The severe nutritional deficiency causes a multitude of problems that must be addressed medically and which make response to medication treatment alone poor. Indeed, no medication has shown significant consistent benefit in the treatment of anorexia. One theory holds that patients with anorexia become addicted to starvation; it is known that endorphins are released during prolonged fasting. This theory holds that anorectics have a biological vulnerability to becoming addicted to fasting. Studies have shown some benefit of naltrexone (an opiate antagonist) in the treatment of anorexia—the explanation being that it blocks the "high" of fasting and thereby removes the incentive (Luby, Marrazzi, and Kinzie 1987). Other medications *sometimes* helpful include antidepressants, antipsychotics, cyproheptadine, and lithium (see figure 13-A). These drugs can be especially useful when there are coexisting features, for instance antidepressants when depressive features are present.

Bulimia, in contrast, often benefits from treatment with antidepressants (40 to 70 percent respond) and is considered by some to be a depressive variant. All types

---

Medications for Treating Eating Disorders

Disorder	Medication
Anorexia	Naloxone/naltrexone
	Antidepressants
	Antipsychotics
	Cyproheptadine
	Lithium
Bulimia	Antidepressants (SSRIs, TCAs, or MAOIs)

Figure 13-A

of antidepressants have proven useful, although it should be remembered that bupropion (Wellbutrin) is contraindicated in eating disorders because of increased incidence of convulsions. Selective serotonin reuptake inhibitors (SSRIs) have been quite effective and, because of their low side effect profile, are often tried first.

Attention Deficit Disorder

Attention deficit disorder first manifests itself in childhood, usually during the first few years of school. It has been called hyperactivity and minimal brain dysfunction in the past. The central feature is a difficulty focusing attention on anything for more than a brief time. This often leads to impulsive behavior and difficulty learning in school. As defined in the *DSM-IV*, attention-deficit/hyperactivity disorder is demonstrated by a patient's meeting the criteria for either inattention or hyperactivity. Inattention is defined as at least six of the following symptoms persisting to a significant degree for at least six months:

Inattention

- Carelessness

- Difficulty sustaining attention

- Not listening

- Failure to follow through on tasks

- Difficulty with organizing activities

- Avoidance of activities requiring prolonged mental effort

- Forgetfulness

- Frequent distraction

- Frequent loss of materials required for activities

Hyperactivity-impulsivity is defined as at least four of the following symptoms persisting to a significant degree for at least six months:

Hyperactivity

- Fidgeting or squirming

- Leaving seat in class

- Inappropriate activity—running, climbing

- Difficulty playing quietly

Impulsivity

- Answering questions before they are completely stated

- Difficulty waiting for turn

Additional criteria for ADD are onset by age 7, symptoms present in two or more situations, and that the behavior causes significant distress or impairment.

Attention Deficit Disorder is thought to have a neurological basis, as implied in the name "minimal brain dysfunction." That name was dropped because the exact "dysfunction" could not be proven and "soft" (equivocal) neurological signs are not always present. Attention deficit disorder has been shown to have significant comorbidity with conduct disorder, depression, bipolar disorder, anxiety disorders, mental retardation, Tourette's syndrome, and borderline personality disorder. It was previously thought that all kids with ADD "grew out of it" during adolescence. Recently, however, a syndrome called residual ADD has been described. This term refers to a persistence of symptoms of ADD into adulthood and is associated with significant impairment, for example, in work performance. Approximately 70 percent of children with ADD go on to experience ADD symptoms in adolescence and adulthood.

Medications play an important part in the treatment of ADD. Stimulants are the mainstay of the treatment of ADD: methylphenidate (Ritalin), dextroamphetamine (Dexedrine), and pemoline (Cylert). These differ in their half-lives, with Ritalin having the shortest and Cylert the longest. There is individual variability in response, so that a person who does not respond to one may respond well to another. Other medications can also be effective in the treatment of ADD and may be useful, especially in residual ADD, where substance abuse may be an issue. These include tricyclic antidepressants (especially desipramine and imipramine) SSRIs, bupropion, and clonidine. There are reports of antipsychotics and lithium being helpful in selected cases, as well.

Self-Mutilation

Self-mutilation refers to deliberate self-injury without the intent to die. It is most commonly encountered in three groups of patients: those with organic disorders (including mental retardation), psychotic disorders, and personality disorders. Self-mutilation is often a clinical issue in patients with severe personality disorders who, for example, repeatedly make lacerations (often fairly superficial) on their wrist or forearm. They may describe feeling that, as they watch the blood flow from the cut, it feels as if some internal tension is flowing out of them.

Recently, there has been growing interest into the possible biological substrate of this type of behavior. Studies have involved the opiate, dopamine, and serotonin systems. It has been shown that endorphins (endogenous opiates) are released by painful stimulation. Opiate antagonists (such as naltrexone) have been helpful in reducing self-injurious behavior (Winchel and Stanley 1991). Self-injurious behavior in animals has been increased by dopamine agonists and decreased by dopamine blockers. Serotonin has also been implicated, partly by the similarity between self-mutilation and some behaviors seen in obsessive-compulsive disorder—irresistible urges to commit an act and the resulting relief from anxiety that follows commission. Selective serotonin re-uptake inhibitors have been shown to be helpful in treating trichotillomania (hair pulling).

A wide variety of medications have been found to sometimes be helpful in self-injurious behavior. Those that have been found to sometimes be helpful in self-injurious behavior in the context of a personality disorder, including MAO inhibitors, SSRIs, carbamazepine, lithium, antipsychotics, and benzodiazepines. The choice of medication should be based on the associated features present. Thus, when depressive features are present, try an SSRI; when there are symptoms of atypical depression and rejection sensitivity, an MAOI; and when psychotic features are present, an antipsychotic. This is an area where there are no clear guidelines for medication use and no guarantee of effectiveness. However, using trial and error, one can often find a drug that has significant benefit.

Part Three

Medications

Part three deals with the different classes of psychopharmaceuticals, including dosage and choice of medication, side effects, and mechanism of action (where and in so far as it has been established). Also covered are precautions for monitoring medication effects and serum levels, and guidelines for educating patients and their families about the effects and side effects of these drugs.

14

Antidepressant Medications

The term *antidepressants* refers to a large, important group of medications used to treat depression. In recent years, they have grown enormously in frequency of prescription and populatory, as well as notoriety. This growth is due to increased awareness of depression and decreased troublesome side effects from the newer agents.

Antidepressants were developed in the 1950s. Iproniazid, an agent used to treat tuberculosis, was inadvertently found to produce an improvement in mood. Ultimately, it was discovered to be an inhibitor of monoamine oxidase (MAO)—an enzyme used to break down catecholamines (dopamine, norepinephrine, and serotonin) in neurons. This led to the development of an entire class of antidepressants: the monoamine oxidase inhibitors or MAOIs.

At about the same time, the drug imipramine was first produced. It was originally developed as a phenothiazine (antipsychotic), but was found to have antidepressant properties. Soon came amitriptyline, followed later by other "tricyclic" and "heterocyclic" antidepressants.

We now have at least three major groups of antidepressants: cyclic antidepressants, selective serotonin reuptake inhibitors (SSRIs), and MAO inhibitors. Additionally, stimulants (such as Dexedrine, Ritalin), atypical antidepressants (bupropion and venlafaxine) and buspirone have been used to treat depression.

Types of Antidepressant Drugs

Tricyclics

For many years, tricyclic antidepressants (TCAs) and heterocyclics have been the mainstay of the treatment of severe depression. The following is a list with their brand names:

Cyclic Antidepressants	
Generic Name	**Brand Name**
Amitriptyline	Elavil
Amoxapine	Asendin
Clomipramine	Anafranil
Desipramine	Norpramin, Pertofrane
Doxepin	Sinequan, Adapin
Imipramine	Tofranil
Maprotiline	Ludiomil
Nortriptyline	Pamelor, Aventyl
Protriptyline	Vivactil
Trazodone	Desyrel
Trimipramine	Surmontil

No antidepressant has been proven consistently superior to another but they do differ significantly in terms of side effects. All of the tricyclics have the same side effects, but in varying degrees. These side effects can be grouped as follows:

- Anticholinergic
- Adrenergic
- Antihistaminic
- Miscellaneous

The tricyclics are considered "dirty" drugs in that they react with a number of receptors besides the one responsible for the therapeutic effect, resulting in a host of side effects (see figure 14-A). Anticholinergic side effects range from unpleasant (dry mouth, dry skin, blurred vision, and constipation) to serious (paralytic ileus, cessation of movement of the intestine, which can lead to intestinal rupture and death; and urinary retention, inability to urinate, which in serious cases can lead to rupture of the bladder). Adrenergic side effects include sweating, sexual dysfunction, and orthostatic hypotension—sudden drop in the blood pressure upon rising and a sensation of lightheadedness. This condition can lead to a fall and, in turn, to fractures, which can have serious medical consequences, especially in the elderly. Antihistaminic effects include sedation and weight gain. Miscellaneous side effects include lowered seizure threshold, cardiac arrhythmia, hepatitis, agranulocytosis, rashes, sweating, anxiety, and elevated heart rate.

Side Effects of Cyclic Antidepressants

	Anticholinergic	Sedation	Orthostatic
Amitriptyline	+++	+++	+++
Amoxapine	++	++	++
Clomipramine	++	++	++
Desipramine	+	±	+
Doxepin	+++	+++	+++
Imipramine	++	++	++
Maprotiline	++	+++	+++
Nortriptyline	+	+	+
Protripyline	+++	++	++
Trazodone	+	++	++
Trimipramine	+++	+++	+++

Figure 14-A

Selective Serotonin Re-uptake Inhibitors

The SSRIs are a newer class of antidepressants. They have been used widely because they are as effective as the tricyclics, but have significantly fewer side effects and are safer in overdosage. The first SSRI on the market was fluoxetine (Prozac). Two newer agents are sertraline (Zoloft) and paroxetine (Paxil), and another agent will soon be available, fluvoxamine. They share the same side effects but in varying degrees (see figure 14-B). Unlike the tricyclics, they are relatively "clean," and interact very little with other receptors besides the serotonin 5-HT re-uptake receptor. Their side effects tend to be related to increased serotonin activity: nausea, gastrointestinal upset, sweating, anxiety, insomnia, headache, restlessness, and sexual dysfunction. They can have mild anticholinergic side effects and can cause dry mouth, sedation, and blurred vision. Such side effects generally are considerably less than those seen with cyclic antidepressants.

Side Effects of SSRI Antidepressants

	Anxiety	Sedation	Insomnia	Nausea
Fluoxetine	++	±	++	+
Paroxetine	±	++	±	+
Sertraline	+	+	+	++

Figure 14-B

Another difference between the SSRI antidepressants is their half-lives. Paroxetine has a half-life of approximately one day, sertraline one to two days, and fluoxetine seven to ten days. A long half-life is an advantage in maintaining a stable blood level buy a disadvantage when starting or stopping the mediciaton. It takes six weeks to reach a steady state with fluoxetine.

Monoamine Oxidase Inhibitors

The MAO inhibitors represent a group of antidepressants now used mainly when other antidepressants have failed for atypical depression, and panic disorder. This is partly because of the risk of a hypertensive reaction. The MAOIs can cause a severe and sudden rise in blood pressure, potentially leading to cerebral hemorrhage or death. Such a reaction can be caused by eating foods high in tyramine content (see figure 14-C) or taking sympathomimetic drugs, such as decongestants or other antidepressants.[1] Thus, it is recommended that people taking MAOIs wear a medic alert bracelet and carry with them nifedipine, an antidote for the hypertensive reaction. In one study of 182 people taking MAOIs, 12 hypertensive reactions occurred, with no fatalities, giving a rate of about 7 percent (Rabkin et al. 1985). In addition to the hypertensive reactions, which are fortunately uncommon, there are a number of other side effects that can be troublesome. These include sedation, insomnia, agitation, confusion, orthostatic symptoms, and edema.

Phenelzine (Nardil), tranylcypromine (Parnate), and isocarboxazid (Marplan) are the three most common MAOIs. Two newer MAOIs are being studied to evaluate their clinical use; both have a reduced risk of hypertensive reaction. Selegiline (Deprenyl) is an MAO-A inhibitor (inhibits type A MAO) that is used in the treatment of Parkinson's disease and may be especially useful for treating depression in patients with Parkinson's. Meclobemide, a reversible MAO-B inhibitor, is currently used in Europe and may soon be available in this country.

Atypical Antidepressants

Bupropion is a relatively new antidepressant with unique properties. It is weakly serotonergic and dopaminergic. It has side effects of anxiety and insomnia. It has received much attention because of its tendency to lower the seizure threshold, having caused convulsions in several patients with eating disorders. Because of this, it is contraindicated for patients with eating disorders, a history of seizures, or patients at risk for seizures (such as those in alcohol withdrawal). However, further evidence indicates the risk of seizures is only slightly higher than the risk with tricyclic antidepressants (4 to 5 per 1000 versus 2 or 3 per 1000). Bupropion has been shown to be effective in patients who failed to respond to tricyclics or SSRIs.

Venlafaxine (Effexor) is a new antidepressant that has recently become available. It has been studied in the treatment of people who did not benefit from other antidepressants ("treatment-resistant"). Usual side effects from venlafaxine are nausea, sedation, and possible dry mouth, dizziness, blurred vision, and anxiety.

Buspirone (BuSpar) is a medication used mainly for the treatment of anxiety. However, there are several reports of its effectiveness as an antidepressant in higher

---

1. In a study by Bieck and Antonin (1988) 50 percent of patients taking tranylcypromine (Parnate) showed a significant hypertensive reaction from taking 8 mg of tyramine.

Tyramine Contents in Food Products

Food	Tyramine Content per Serving
Fish	
Lumpfish roe	0.2 mg/50 g
Sliced schmaltz herrring in oil	0.2 mg/50 g
Pickled herring[a]	negligible
Smoked salmon	negligible
Salmon mousse	0.7 mg/30 g
Meat and sausage	
Salami	5.6 mg/30 g
Mortadella	5.5 mg/30 g
Air-dried sausage	3.8 mg/30 g
Chicken liver	1.5 mg/30 g
Bologna	1.0 mg/30 g
Aged sausage	0.9 mg/30 g
Smoked meat	0.5 mg/30 g
Corned beef	0.3 mg/30 g
Kielbasa sausage	0.2 mg/30 g
Fruit	
Avocado[a]	negligible
Banana[a]	negligible
Banana peel	1.424 mg/banana
Raisins[a]	negligible
Figs[a]	negligible
Other	
Marmite concentrated yeast extract	6.45 mg/10 g
Sauerkraut	13.87 mg
Beef bouillon mix	231.25 µg/package
Beef bouillon	102.00 µg/cube
Soy sauce	0.2 mg/10 ml
Yogurt[a]	negligible
Fava beans[a]	negligible
Beer	0.3–1.5 mg
Wine	0–0.5 mg

[a] Previously thought to be higher in tyramine
Source: Shulman et al. 1989.

Figure 14-C

doses (40–60 mg per day and up). It has the side effects of anxiety (paradoxically), nausea, headache, and dizziness.

Stimulants

Stimulants have been used as antidepressants for many years, especially dextroamphetamine (Dexedrine) and methylphenidate (Ritalin). They have the side effects of anxiety, insomnia, agitation, and appetite suppression. They can be quite effective antidepressants but are now usually reserved for medically ill patients such as those who have had a stroke and those unresponsive to other antidepressants.

Mechanism of Action

The antidepressants, generally, produce their therapeutic effects by blocking the reuptake of one or more catecholamines (norepinephrine, serotonin, and dopamine), which leads to a decrease (down-regulation) of the number of post-synaptic receptors—generally within seven to twenty-one days, coinciding with the onset of clinical effect (see chapter 3). The MAOIs block monoamine oxidase, which metabolizes the catecholamines stored at the nerve ending of the presynaptic neuron—thereby making more catecholamine available. Stimulants increase the release of catecholamines. Buspirone is a 5-HT IA receptor blocker.

Antidepressants generally produce effects within two to three weeks. Once therapeutic benefit has been obtained, it is important that the patient continue the medication for at least six months. Discontinuing in less than six months is likely to lead to relapse. In treating a patient's first depression, it is reasonable to gradually discontinue the medication after six to twelve months. If the patient has had two or more depressions, it is probably best to continue the medication because the likelihood of recurrence is significant (70 to 80 percent or more). Recent studies have also shown that subsequent depressive episodes may be less responsive to treatment. Therefore, in such cases the best treatment is to prevent relapse by continuation of medication.

Dosages

In order for medications to be effective, they must be taken at an adequate dose (see figure 14-D). There seems to be a threshold effect, with subtherapeutic doses producing little or no benefit. However, achieving effective doses may be difficult due to the side effects of tricyclic antidepressants and MAOIs. Blood levels may be helpful to check the adequacy of tricylic dosage (see figure 14-E).

Nortriptyline appears to be the one antidepressant that has a bell-shaped response curve (or therapeutic window): both doses too low and too high are less effective. Thus blood levels can be very helpful when using nortriptyline. For other antidepressants, blood levels may be helpful to see if the dose needs to be increased. Usually antidepressants are started at a low dose, for example, fluoxetine at 10–20 mg or desipramine at 10–25 mg, and titrated upward. This is because of the wide variability (greater than tenfold) in absorption of these medicaitons.

Initially, you will see only side effects. Over the course of one to two weeks, tolerance usually develops to the side effects, and the dose can be increased into the therapeutic range. Some people will sleep for one or more full days after taking a single dose of a sedating antidepressant, and afterwards may be reluctant to take any antidepressant. Such incidents and other side effects can be avoided by starting the patient at a low dose and increasing it slowly.

Other side effects are often easily managed. Dry mouth is common with tricyclics and can be managed by drinking water, chewing gum, or using synthetic saliva (available at a pharmacy). Constipation can be managed with a stool softener (such as Metamucil or DSS). Orthostatic symptoms can be managed by avoiding dehydration, standing up gradually, and holding onto something for a few seconds after standing. For the SSRIs, nausea often can be managed by taking the medication with a meal. Insomnia may require taking the medication only in the morning and sometimes by taking a sedating medication at bedtime. Anxiety can be reduced by avoiding caffeine and phenylpropanolamine (and other decongestants). Sexual dysfunction can often be improved by using the medication cyproheptadine. (Many more measures can be taken to manage other side effects, but they are beyond the scope of this book.)

Antidepressant Doses

Drug	Dose (mg/day)
Cyclics	
Amitriptyline	75–300
Doxepin	75–300
Imipramine	75–300
Trimipramine	75–300
Clomipramine	75–200
Amoxapine	150–400
Desipramine	75–300
Maprotiline	75–225
Nortriptyline	50–150
Protriptyline	15–60
Trazodone	150–400
SSRIs	
Fluoxetine	20–80
Sertraline	50–200
Paroxetine	20–60
MAOIs	
Phenelzine	45–90
Tranylcypromine	20–40
Isocarboxazid	20–30

Figure 14-D

Blood Levels of Cyclic Antidepressants	
Drug	**Typical Plasma Concentration (mg/ml)**
Amitriptyline	100–250
Doxepin	100–250
Imipramine	200–300
Trimipramine	250–300
Clomipramine	200–300
Amoxapine	150–500
Desipramine	100–250
Maprotiline	250–300
Nortriptyline	50–150
Protriptyline	100–250
Trazodone	800–1600

Figure 14-E

When these measures do not work and the patient complains of troublesome or intolerable side effects, one can decrease the dosage (which may lead to a loss of benefit) or change to another medication, as is addressed in the next section.

Choice of Medication

Probably the two most important considerations for choosing a medication are the patient's previous response to antidepressants and his or her family history of response to antidepressants. All the antidepressants are statistically equivalent in their effectiveness. One has not been proven consistently superior; some work for some people and others work for other people. There is no means to know beforehand which medication an individual will respond to. So the best choice is to use a medication that the patient or a biological relative has responded to in the past.

The next best choice is based on minimizing undesirable side effects. Thus, a patient complains of anxiety and insomnia, you might use a sedating medication. Or, conversely, if the individual complains of lack of energy, you might choose a nonsedating or energizing antidepressant. Many professionals feel that because of their safety, efficacy, and lack of side effects that the SSRIs are the first choice in the treatment of depression. Others continue to prescribe TCAs first because of their long record of efficacy and lower cost. Many clinicians prefer the secondary amines (refers to chemical structure) over the tertiary amine tricyclics, because they have fewer side effects. The secondary amines are amoxapine, desipramine, maprotiline, nortriptyline, and protriptyline.

Whichever antidepressant is chosen first, the question of what to try if the first one doesn't work may arise. But what is considered a nonresponse? Before you abandon one medication for another, it is important that the patient experience an "adequate clinical trial." This means adequate time at an adequate dose—at least four weeks, and some studies suggest eight to twelve weeks because there is a small percentage of late responders. But then, what is an adequate dose—the usual dose, such as 200 mg of imipramine, or the maximum tolerated dose? (Again, blood levels may help.) Medication compliance must also be considered.

When switching, it probably makes sense to try an antidepressant quite different from the first. For example, if the first was serotonergic, try one that is noradrenergic (or vice versa). Some people suggest that it makes sense to try one noradrenergic, one SSRI, and one dopaminergic antidepressant (see figure 14-F). Special considerations also apply to certain classes of patients when selecting an antidepressant—see figure 14-G.

Treatment-Resistant Depression

Much has been written about "treatment-resistant" depression. *Treatment-resistant depression* (TRD) refers to a depression that has failed to respond to adequate trials of two or more antidepressants. As many as 30 percent of people with depression may fall into this category—although it probably is closer to 10 to 20 percent.

Generic Name	Norepinephrine Effects	Serotonin Effects	Monoamine Oxidase Effects	Dopamine Effects
Imipramine	++	+++	0	0
Desipramine	+++++	0	0	0
Amitriptyline	+	++++	0	0
Nortriptyline	+++	++	0	0
Protriptyline[a]	++++	+	0	0
Trimipramine[a]	++	++	0	0
Doxepin[a]	+++	++	0	0
Maprotiline	+++++	0	0	0
Amoxapine	++++	+	0	0
Venlafaxine	++	+++	0	+
Trazodone	0	+++++	0	0
Fluoxetine	0	+++++	0	0
Paroxetine	0	+++++	0	0
Sertraline	0	+++++	0	0
Bupropion[b]	±	±	0	+
Phenelzine	0	0	+++++	0
Tranylcypromine	0	0	+++++	0
Isocarboxazid	0	0	+++++	0

Table title: **Selective Action of Antidepressant Medications**

[a] Uncertain, but likely effects
[b] Atypical antidepressant; uncertain effects but likely to be a dopamine and norepinephrine agonist

Figure 14-F

A full discussion of the treatment of TRD is beyond the scope of this book, but it will be helpful for you to be familiar with some of the typical strategies used in such cases. The following list should be considered in the treatment of resistant depression, but is by no means exhaustive:

- Check the diagnosis: Are depressive symptoms due to characterological disorder, medical illness, or psychotic disorder?

- Is it a type of depression that typically is not responsive to medication treatment (such as psychological-reactive depression), so that psychotherapy is instead the treatment of choice?

- Check the dose: Has the medication dose been too low? (It may help to check the blood level.) Has the patient taken the medication as prescribed and for a long enough period of time (at least four to six weeks at adequate dose)?

- Check for substance abuse, especially alcohol.

- Change the medication: Usually you will want to try another class of medication (NE, 5-HT, MAOI).

- Augmentation: The addition of lithium, thyroid, or a stimulant medication may lead to a positive response. Also, another antidepressant may be added to the current medication: for instance, you might add a serotonergic drug to a noradrenergic, or vice versa. Fluoxetine has been used in this fashion frequently. Note however that this approach necessitates a lowering of the dose of the other antidepressant.

- Consider electroconvulsive treatment.

- Venlafaxine is a new antidepressant, specifically studied for use in treatment-resistant depression, and may be a treatment option.

Special Considerations in Choosing an Antidepressant

Patient Type	Medication Choices
Child	TCA (monitor EKG), possibly SSRI
Elderly	Secondary amine TCA (desipramine, nortriptyline) or SSRI, bupropion
Anxious or agitated	Trazodone consider tertiary amine TCA
Retarded or anergic	SSRI, bupropion, secondary amine TCA
Psychotic	Amoxapine, TCA, possibly SSRI (used with an antipsychotic)
Atypical	MAOI, SSRI
Bipolar	Bupropion (possibly less likely to cause mania) SSRI, TCA, MAOI
High suicide risk	Less toxic antidepressants (fluoxetine, trazodone, paroxetine, sertraline, bupropion, venlafaxine)

Figure 14-G

Patient Education

Education of patients about antidepressants has several facets. First, education about the biological aspects of depression is helpful, especially so that they do not view taking medication as a sign of moral weakness. Next, it is important to describe what to expect from the antidepressants: what typical side effects are, that the medication is not habit forming, that a clinical response typically takes two to three weeks to be achieved, that side effects diminish over time, and that other medications can be tried if the first one does not work. For people taking MAOIs, education about foods and medications to avoid is crucial.

The most common cause of medication failure is failure to take enough medication for long enough. Discussion about side effects can be very helpful in helping someone continue the medication long enough to benefit. This can be difficult, because initially there are only side effects and no benefits; only later are there benefits and diminished side effects. Through supportive therapy you can often help your depressed patient to overcome annoyance or distress over side effects (preoccupation with somatic symptoms), discouragement about delayed benefits, and pessimism about the outcome. In these ways, you can help your client to continue in treatment and achieve greater benefit.

15

Mood Stabilizers

In the treatment of bipolar disorder, the question of *when* to consider medications is not particularly at issue, since pharmacotherapy is the mainstay of treatment. The more important question may be *what* medication will work best in the particular patient. The primary agents to consider are the mood stabilizers: lithium and the anticonvulsants carbamazepine and valproic acid. These drugs are also referred to as *antimanic agents*, which is not entirely accurate since their therapeutic action includes treatment of both manic and depressive symptoms. Routinely, adjunctive agents will be necessary, such as antipsychotics, antidepressants, and antianxiety agents. This chapter mainly deals with the mood stabilizers, although combination regimens are also covered. In clinical practice, the mood stabilizers are indicated primarily for the various states and subtypes of bipolar disorder and cyclothymia. Frequently, they also promote therapeutic gain as adjuncts in the treatment of schizoaffective disorder, schizophrenia, treatment-resistant major depression, and impulse control disorders.

Lithium

The use of lithium in psychiatry has varied historically. In the nineteenth century, lithium salts were employed in the treatment of anxiety, as well as gout and seizures. The importance of lithium's antimanic actions was indirectly discovered, in 1949, with observations that it produced a calming effect in animals. Human testing in agitated or manic patients followed, with encouraging results. However, lithium's use did not gain acceptance in American medicine until 1970, due to safety concerns following reports of toxicity in cardiac patients who were using lithium chloride as a salt substitute. Lithium is now firmly established as a safe and effective treatment for acute mania and for the prevention of manic-depressive episodes, with response rates in typical bipolar disorder estimated at 60 to 80 percent. However, lithium's mechanism of action remains to be identified. Except for mild cognitive and motor slowing in healthy individuals, lithium does not share the sedating or euphoriant properties of other psychotropics.

Lithium is the lightest of the solid elements, is widely found in nature, and because of its chemical activity will combine with other ions to form lithium salts (Gennaro 1980). Lithium salts share some, but not all, properties of sodium and potassium. The two therapeutically available forms are lithium carbonate and lithium citrate (see figure 15-A).

Available Forms of Lithium

- Lithium carbonate capsules—300 mg available from various manufacturers. Brand names include Eskalith and Lithonate. Only one generic manufacturer currently makes lithium carbonate in 150 mg and 600 mg capsules.

- Lithium carbonate tablets—300 mg available from various manufacturers. Brand names include Eskalith, Lithane, and Lithotabs. Eskalith-CR 450 mg long-acting tablets are also available.

- Lithium citrate—available from various manufacturers. Brand names include Cibalith-S.

Figure 15-A

Lithium demonstrates a narrow *therapeutic window*—the therapeutic dose is very close to the toxic dose. (See also "Therapeutic Index" in appendix A.) Consequently, lithium is prescribed not only by dose, and stage of symptoms, but by concentration in the blood (see figure 15-B). Side effects are often indicative of blood level but not always. During acute states, daily doses of 1200 mg to 2400 mg of lithium are required, with most patients needing less after stabilization (600 to 1800 mg per day). Also, as the acute episode resolves, many patients will become more intolerant of side effects, necessitating a dosage reduction. The onset of action of lithium occurs in five to fourteen days, although full stabilization may take up to several months.

Dosage Guidelines for Lithium

Stage	Dosage Range (mg/day)	Serum Level (mEq/l)
Acute mania	1200–2400	0.8–1.5
Maintenance	600–1800	0.6–1.2

Figure 15-B

Side Effects and Their Management

Lithium produces a distinct continuum of side effects which range from relatively benign, transient symptoms to toxicity that can be fatal. The most significant side effects fall into the following categories.

Gastrointestinal

Nausea, vomiting, and diarrhea can occur to varying degrees at any time during treatment. These side effects may appear at the beginning of treatment or upon dosage increases. *However, GI symptoms may also be one of the critical indicators of lithium toxicity.* Obtaining a lithium blood level in response to the appearance of these symptoms is important. After ruling out an elevated lithium level as a cause of GI symptoms, changing from one dosage form to another, especially to a long-acting or liquid preparation, is often helpful. Lithium may also be administered after meals or the total daily dosage may be divided into smaller doses to alleviate the nausea.

Nervous system and neuromuscular

Initial complaints, which usually diminish with time, include headache, lethargy, and muscle weakness. Nearly half of patients experience a fine hand tremor at some time during lithium treatment. For most people, this initial symptom remits; however, for 10 percent of patients, it is a continuing side effect (American Society of Hospital Pharmacists 1993). Often the tremor becomes worse when the individual reaches for something. Sustained tremor, at therapeutic levels, can be managed with reassurance, and by limiting stimulants, such as caffeine, which may exacerbate the tremor. Sometimes this tremor is treated with beta blockers, usually propranolol (Inderal).

Not all neurologic side effects are benign; sometimes they are indicators of toxicity. *Worsening of tremor, confusion, stupor, and slurred speech are warning signs that require a lithium blood level to be taken to rule out toxicity.* Severe lithium toxicity can result in seizures, CNS depression, irregular heartbeat, decreased kidney function, coma, or death. Although various emergency measures, including dialysis, can be employed in lithium intoxication, there is no antidote. An episode of severe lithium intoxication will resolve as the drug is eliminated from the body, usually over several days. A small number of patients are left with permanent neurological impairment following acute or chronic dosage excesses.

Endocrine

Thyroid hormones are frequently affected by lithium, but rarely in a clinically significant way. Changes in certain laboratory tests of thyroid function are common but seldom require discontinuation of treatment. However, approximately 5 percent of patients develop hypothyroidism, which some clinicians elect to treat with thyroid supplementation while continuing lithium (Weber, Saklad, and Kastenhol 1992). Periodic thyroid function monitoring is important, not only from a safety standpoint but to rule out (in the bipolar individual with depressed or mixed-state features), that hypothyroidism is not the cause of symptoms.

Renal

The pharmacokinetics of lithium are important in understanding its kidney-related side effects. Lithium, unlike most other medications, relies only on the kidney for elimination from the body, without any liver metabolism. Therefore, adequate kidney function is critical to safe lithium use. *Interference or alteration in normal kidney functioning can potentially lead to a buildup of lithium.* Lithium use usually should be avoided in the presence of renal disease. Also, since elderly people in general show age-related decreases in kidney function, lithium should be prescribed cautiously and with appropriately reduced dosages.

Additionally, lithium excretion is directly related, in an *inverse* way, to sodium excretion. Conditions leading to excess sodium elimination will cause a corresponding increase in the amount of lithium retained in the body. Excessive sodium loss occurs from diarrhea, vomiting, fever, dehydration, profuse sweating, diuretic medications, and severely salt-restricted diets.

The benign effects of lithium on the kidney will be experienced by the majority of patients as increased thirst (polydipsia) and increased urination (polyuria). To ensure adequate lithium excretion, patients must be advised to maintain fluid intake, even in the presence of polyuria.

Since the late 1970s, debate concerning potential long-term kidney damage with lithium has continued. It is now generally accepted that minor structural changes can be demonstrated in about 10 percent of lithium-treated patients (*Facts and Comparisons* 1993). However, such changes have also been reported in bipolar populations before lithium therapy. Additionally, these changes do not necessarily mean impairment in overall kidney function, although lithium intoxication can cause at least time-limited alterations in kidney structure.

Hematological

A benign, reversible increase in white blood cell (WBC) count occurs frequently with lithium treatment. This is clinically nonsignificant and does not require discontinuation of treatment.

Cardiovascular

It is not unusual for lithium to induce some minor changes on electrocardiogram (EKG) studies. However, serious cardiac problems are rare at therapeutic levels.

Dermatological

The more common dermatological effects of lithium treatment are rash and acne-like lesions. Whether to stop lithium therapy is determined by the severity of either of these conditions.

Weight gain

Various mechanisms have been proposed, without conclusion, for this relatively common side effect, estimated at up to 20 pounds in at least 20 percent of patients. (Vestergaard, Amdisen, and Schow 1980). Supervised caloric restriction may be helpful.

Teratogenicity

Lithium is contraindicated during pregnancy, especially the first trimester, due to congenital abnormalities, most notably of the heart. In rare situations, it may be necessary to continue lithium treatment in the pregnant patient, with dosage adjustments as necessitated by pregnancy-induced changes in kidney function.

Monitoring blood levels

Laboratory monitoring is necessary throughout lithium treatment to determine a safe and therapeutic dose and to limit side effects. The especially critical times to obtain a lithium level are during initiation, with dosage changes, with breakthrough

Recommended Lithium Monitoring

Reason	Frequency
Initiation of treatment	Every 3 to 7 days for first several weeks
	Once monthly for 3 to 6 months
Routine	Every 1 to 3 months in stable patient
With dosage change	Within 3 to 5 days
Signs of toxicity	Immediate
Symptoms of mania or depression	Immediate
Addition or discontinuation of interacting meds	Within 3 to 5 days
In presence of medical conditions resulting in dehydration	Immediate
Suspected pregnancy	Immediate

Figure 15-C

symptoms, and any time toxicity is suspected (see figure 15-C). In the presence of severe side effects the prescriber will often discontinue lithium, pending laboratory results. Even though side effects and serum levels are not absolutely correlated in all patients, there is a general association (in figure 15-D).

Mechanism of Action

Decades of research have yet to provide a clear understanding of the exact mechanism of action of lithium. Multiple sites of action within the CNS have been identified, none of which fully explain lithium's action on both mania and depression. Since neurotransmitter production, release, and re-uptake rely on various ions (sodium, calcium, potassium, and magnesium), lithium's ionic properties may affect neurotransmitter-mediated depression and mania. Another potential mechanism of

Severity of Side Effects

Mild	Moderate	Severe
(Lithium level up to 1.5)	(Lithium level 1.5–2.5)	(Lithium level above 2.5)
Increased thirst	Recurring, persisting or worsening nausea, vomiting or diarrhea	Decreased urine output
Increased urination		Stupor
Weight gain		Seizure
Nausea, vomiting diarrhea	Coarse tremor	Cardiovascular collapse
Fine hand tremor	Muscle twitching	Coma, death
Muscle weakness	Confusion	
Drowsiness	Slurred speech	
Lethargy		

Figure 15-D

action of lithium is linked to its ability to stabilize cell membranes, via activity at sodium and potassium channels.

Lithium's benefit in mania may be linked to effects on dopamine and norepinephrine, possibly by preventing dopamine receptor supersensitivity in the manic individual. Additionally, lithium blocks some cocaine- and amphetamine-induced symptoms of mania, which are thought to be mediated by stimulant-related increases in CNS dopamine concentration. The action of lithium on norepinephrine is variable, causing an initial prolonged increase in reuptake, although this effect is not evident with long-term administration (American Society of Hospital Pharmacists 1993).

Lithium's serotonergic activity is postulated to be responsible for its role in preventing depressive episodes of bipolar disorder. Some bipolar patients demonstrate low CNS concentrations of serotonin. Lithium may contribute to serotonin production by increasing the uptake of the tryptophan, a serotonin precursor (American Society of Hospital Pharmacists 1993).

Current research strongly suggests that lithium's actions *inside* neuronal cells explain therapeutic effects (Weber, Saklad, and Kastenholz 1992). Specifically, lithium inhibits receptor-induced overactivity of intracellular secondary messenger systems. These secondary messengers can be sent into overactive cycles by the action of various neurotransmitters at the receptor. Some neurotransmitters may induce manic symptoms; others may induce depressive symptoms. Lithium's ability to interrupt these overactive pathways, regardless of the triggering neurotransmitter, may explain its action in both depression and mania.

Anticonvulsants

Two anticonvulsants, carbamazepine (Tegretol) and valproic acid, also referred to as valproate (Depakote, Depakene), have proven mood-stabilizing properties (see figure 15-E). These agents are most useful when lithium is contraindicated or when a patient does not respond to or cannot tolerate lithium. Rapid cyclers, who often are poorly controlled with lithium, are good candidates for one of these alternative agents. Valproic acid appears to be indicated more for manic or mixed states of bipolar disorder, and is probably not as effective in depressed states. The anticonvulsants are often employed in conjunction with lithium.

Like lithium, exact mechanisms of action have yet to be identified for the anticonvulsants. Carbamazepine, which is chemically related to tricyclic antidepressants, has been used to treat bipolar disorder since the 1970s. However, its actions as an anticonvulsant have been more widely studied than its antimanic properties. The kindling process may provide an explanation of carbamazepine's functioning. Explored for its potential in the pathogenesis of both affective disorders and seizure disorders, the kindling theory suggests that subthreshold stimuli to certain brain areas ultimately produces specific activity—psychiatric or behavioral manifestations or seizure activity. This model attempts to demonstrate a common substrate based on neurologic and episodic similarities. The discovery of the mood-stabilizing properties of the anticonvulsants contributed to interest in this area of inquiry.

While it is tempting to hypothesize that this association exists, the theory remains unproven—as does the exact mechanism of carbamazepine's dual action in these disorders. The lack of an adequate biological model for the pathogenesis of bipolar disorder adds to the difficulty of drawing conclusions about carbamazepine's actions.

Available Forms of Anticonvulsants

- Carbamazepine—200 mg tablets, 100 mg chewable tablets, 100 mg/tsp liquid. Brand names include Tegretol.

- Valproic acid—125 mg, 250 mg, 500 mg delayed-release tablets; 125 mg and 250 mg capsules; 250 mg/tsp liquid. Brand names include Depakote and Depakene.

Figure15-E

Dosage Guidelines for Anticonvulsants

Drug	Dosage Range[a] (mg / day)	Serum Level[b] (mcg / ml)
Carbamazepine	600–1600	4–10+
Valproic acid	750–1500	50–100

[a] Serum levels are based on established anticonvulsant use. Mood-stabilizing response may fall above or below these values

[b] Dosage requirements may be less for patients on multiple psychotropics.

Figure 15-F

Side Effects and Their Management

There are important therapeutic and side effect differences between carbamazepine and valproic acid. Side effects are experienced by about 30 percent of patients treated with carbamazepine (Hollister 1992). Central nervous system effects are common, and include sedation, dizziness, drowsiness, blurred vision, and incoordination. Gastrointestinal side effects include nausea, vomiting, diarrhea, and abdominal pain, all of which may be alleviated by taking the medication with food or milk. Many of the CNS and GI side effects are often dose related and can be minimized by small dosage increases during titration or dosage reduction. Dermatological side effects can manifest with a red, itching rash or hives; they often necessitate discontinuation of treatment.

Carbamazepine can induce decreases in white blood cell (WBC) count. These changes may be slight, especially during the first few weeks of treatment, and do not absolutely warrant stopping the medication. However, with a significant reduction in WBC or related components, most clinicians will consider discontinuing the medication and further evaluate these hematological changes.

Valproic acid is tolerated slightly better than carbamazepine relative to nervous system side effects, notably in fewer complaints of fatigue and dizziness. Gastrointestinal side effects of nausea, vomiting, and indigestion, are common, although these are usually transient. Use of sustained-release tablets (Depakote) may reduce these effects. Valproic acid can occasionally interfere with the normal blood clotting cycle. Potential liver damage is also possible with valproate, although this effect has primarily been demonstrated in children taking multiple anticonvulsant medications.

Blood level monitoring is required for carbamazepine and valproic acid, utilizing therapeutic anticonvulsant ranges (see figure 15-F). While there are not established ranges for antimanic effects, performing routine monitoring will identify potentially toxic levels. Levels should be taken weekly for the first month and every one to three months thereafter. Excessively elevated serum levels (overdoses) of the anticonvulsants are potentially life-threatening. Associated with carbamazepine toxicity are neurologic and cardiac malfunctions, while valproic acid overdose may produce somnolence and coma.

Mechanism of Action

Carbamazepine continues to be studied with regard to its actions on primary and secondary neurotransmitter systems and on sodium and potassium ion channels. It has a limited ability to block norepinephrine reuptake (Hollister 1992) and has been reported to decrease norepinephrine release (Post, Weiss, and Chuang 1992). Dopamine release is enhanced, and reuptake is blocked. As with lithium and valproate, long-term administration causes an increase in GABA receptors (upregulation) in the hippocampus, but not in the cortex (Post, Weiss, and Chuang 1992).

Even though valproic acid shares with carbamazepine many of the properties described above, the more likely mechanism of valproate in bipolar disorder is through increased GABA levels in the CNS.

Combinations of Medication

Patients with bipolar disorder frequently require multiple medications or changes in therapy. For example, antianxiety agents are helpful in reducing anxiety and agitation, especially in patients who refuse antimanic or antipsychotic agents. Likewise an added antipsychotic is more effective than lithium alone in acute manic episodes that include significant psychomotor activity and delusions or hallucinations. Ongoing treatment with antipsychotics after the manic episode is resolved is often not necessary. However, it is not uncommon for a refractory patient to require a combination of mood stabilizers, an antidepressant, and an antipsychotic.

For the patient with persistent depressive symptoms, antidepressants are often necessary. However, the possibility of triggering a "switch" into mania must always be considered. Some clinicians report less risk with monoamine oxidase inhibitors or bupropion than with tricyclic or serotonin-specific antidepressants.

Length of Treatment

Patients with bipolar disorder face long-term (lifetime) treatment with medications. Although use of antidepressants and antipsychotics may be limited to specific periods, a mood stabilizer is considered routine maintenance therapy in most patients. Medication-free periods are seldom beneficial and often result in symptom relapse.

Patient Education

Comprehensive patient education is critical in ensuring compliance and in ultimately limiting the devastating effects of bipolar disorder. Perhaps the most difficult fact for the patient to accept is the need for long-term treatment. In addition, patients must become active participants in identifying target symptoms and critical side effects, especially with lithium.

The first year after diagnosis can be an extremely difficult time for the patient and is often marked by treatment noncompliance and relapse. Thus patient education should include a discussion of the serious implications of medication noncompliance. Some individuals may naively (or out of denial) view periodic manic episodes as relatively benign occurrences, when in fact these are times of increased mortality risk. Patients should be informed that recurring manic episodes may increase susceptibility to future episodes. Additionally, some patients may actually become less responsive to lithium treatment with repeated episodes of mania. The therapist can be instrumental in helping patients recognize that continued medication noncompliance may actually contribute to a progressive worsening of their disorder.

Psychotherapeutic Issues

Professional opinions about lithium vary by discipline and by individual clinician. Some therapists find it easier to support the use of a "natural" substance, whereas others have been influenced by reports of side effects and toxicity. While the acutely manic patient is most often hospitalized, patients with hypomania or cyclothymia may be initiated on medications as outpatients, making the therapist an important part of the stabilization process. In this role, the therapist can assist the patient in assessing response and identifying side effects.

Patients will often resist mood stabilizers because of concerns not only about side effects but about therapeutic effects. What is clinically considered a symptom may be a desired state for the patient: a higher lever of energy, creativity, confidence. It is important to explore with the patient the sense of loss bipolar patients typically feel when valued conditions are diminished. For the bipolar patient, the desire for the manic "high" can be quite strong, not unlike the craving a drug addict experiences during the initial stages of recovery. This analogy may be helpful to patients who are struggling to accept the disease. The therapist can provide support and reassurance by acknowledging that mania is indeed a powerfully reinforcing "intrinsic high," but eventually the longing to be manic will diminish.

Psychotherapy is not only possible but can be very productive with the bipolar patient. However, the therapist must be skilled at identifying symptoms of hypomania, mania, and depression, and the necessity for medication adjustment referrals. The therapist can be tested especially by the effects of medication noncompliance, when symptoms return and judgment and insight diminish.

16

Antianxiety Medications

The first benzodiazepine synthesized was chlordiazepoxide (Librium), in 1957. Since then, many others have been developed and are available in the United States. These medications are used both for anxiety (sedatives) and insomnia (hypnotics). Additional uses are as anesthetics and as aids in handling withdrawal from other drugs. Some are used primarily as hypnotics (flurazepam, temazepam, and triazolam), but they differ little, other than by use, from the other benzodiazepines. When benzodiazepines were first developed, they represented a significant improvement over the previously available antianxiety agents: the barbiturates, meprobamate (Equanil, Miltown), tybamate (Tybatran), glutethimide (Doriden), methyprylon (Noludar), and ethchlorvynol (Placidyl). The benzodiazepines had better antianxiety specificity and were much less lethal in overdose.

These medications have been very widely used (and abused) because anxiety and insomnia are very common and because these drugs are very effective and well tolerated. Within twenty to thirty minutes after an oral dose the effects can be felt. Benzodiazepines can cause sedation, slurred speech, incoordination, prolonged response time in higher doses (or when the person is very sensitive to the drug), and sometimes a lessening of inhibitions, as with alcohol.

The main differences between the different drugs are their pharmacodynamics: especially half-life and metabolism (see figure 16-A). Those with a longer half-life tend to build up in the system—even if taken only once a day. Most are metabolized by the liver and therefore can build up in the system when the liver is impaired, as with alcoholic liver disease. The three least dependent on the liver are lorazepam, temazepam, and oxazepam. The ones with a very short half-life (triazolam, midazo-

---

Half-Lives of Benzodiazepines

- More than 24 hours:
  Diazepam
  Chlordiazepoxide
  Flurazepam
  Prazepam
  Clorazepate

- 18–24 hours:
  Clonazepam

- 8–16 hours:
  Temazepam
  Lorazepam
  Alprazolam
  Oxazepam

- Less than 6 hours:
  Triazolam
  Midazolam

Figure 16-A

lam, and, to a lesser degree, lorazepam) can cause anterograde amnesia: loss of memory for a short period after the drug has worn off.

Types of Antianxiety Drugs

Benzodiazepines

The benzodiazepines work by interacting with benzodiazepine receptors; of which there are three types. Most current benzodiazepines show little selectivity for these receptor types; however, those developed in the future may have greater selectivity and possibly less sedation or dependence potential. Benzodiazepine receptors are co-located with GABA receptors, which usually function as presynaptic inhibiting receptors. The benzodiazepine receptors have a high density in the limbic system. Binding of a benzodiazepine at the BZ receptor enhances the effect of GABA and increases the influx of chloride ions (see figure 16-B; also see chapter 7 for a more detailed discussion of the biological basis of anxiety disorders). Figure 16-C gives the dosage range for benzodiazepines.

Atypical Benzodiazepines

There are three new benzodiazepine derivatives being used as hypnotics (see figure 16-C). Estazolam (ProSom) is a triazolobenzodiazepine with a rapid onset of action, intermediate half-life, and no significant active metabolites; thus it does not have a tendency to lead to drug accumulation and daytime sedation. Quazepam (Doral) has the same active metabolite as flurazepam and has similar properties. Zolpidem (Ambien) is a short-acting nonbenzodiazepine of the imidazopyridine class. Some studies suggest it may be associated with less cognitive impairment, and less dependence. This may be due to its greater specificity in interacting preferentially with one of the three BZ receptors.

Buspirone

Buspirone is a unique antianxiety agent. It acts at the 5-HT 1A receptor; however, its exact mechanism of action is not fully understood. Buspirone tends to have a delayed onset of action—similar to the antidepressants. A typical starting dose is 5 mg two or three times per day; typically patients require 20–40 mg per day in divided doses (see figure 16-C). Reduced anxiety is seen within one or two weeks.

The advantages of buspirone over benzodiazepines are that it is not associated with tolerance or dependence, it does not interact with other CNS depressants (such as alcohol), and it is not associated with impaired psychomotor function. The drug's disadvantages are its delayed onset of action and that it is not always effective, especially in people who have used benzodiazepines. The most common side effects of buspirone are nausea, dizziness, and, paradoxically, anxiety.

Antihistamines

Certain antihistamines are frequently used in the treatment of anxiety: hydroxyzine (Vistaril, Atarax) and diphenhydramine (Benadryl) (see figure 16-C). They act by blocking histamine receptors in the CNS, causing sedation and thereby reducing anxiety. They can also cause drowsiness and impaired performance. They work

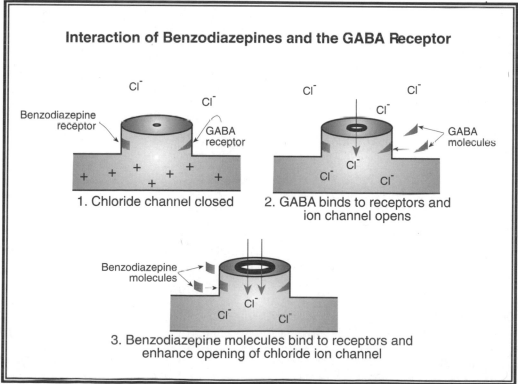

Interaction of Benzodiazepines and the GABA Receptor

1. Chloride channel closed

2. GABA binds to receptors and ion channel opens

3. Benzodiazepine molecules bind to receptors and enhance opening of chloride ion channel

Figure 16-B

within twenty to thirty minutes and last four to six hours. They are not habit-forming, but have the disadvantages that tolerance can develop to their anxiolytic (antianxiety) effects and they tend to have a narrow therapeutic window between reducing anxiety and producing sedation.

Dosages of Antianxiety Agents

Generic Name	Brand Name	Single-Dose Dosage Range (mg)	Usual Dosage Range (mg/day)
Benzodiazepines			
Diazepam	Valium	2–10	4–40
Chlordiazepoxide	Librium	10–50	15–100
Flurazepam	Dalmane	15–60	15–60
Prazepam	Centrax	5–30	20–40
Clorazepate	Tranxene	3.75–15	7.5–60
Clonazepam	Klonopin	0.5–2	1–8
Temazepam	Restoril	15–30	15–60
Lorazepam	Ativan	0.5–2	1.5–6
Alprazolam	Xanax	0.25–2	0.5–6
Oxazepam	Serax	10–30	30–90
Triazolam	Halcion	0.125–0.5	.125–0.5
Midazolam	Versed (injectable only)		
Atypical Benzodiazepines			
Estazolam	ProSom	1.0–2.0	1.0–2.0
Quazepam	Doral	7.5–30	7.5–30
Zolpidem	Ambien	5–10	5–10
Other Antianxiety Agents			
Buspirone	BuSpar	5–20	10–40
Hydroxyzine	Atarax, Vistaril	10–50	30–200
Diphenhydramine	Benadryl	25–100	75–200
Propranolol	Inderal	10–80	20–160
Atenolol	Tenormin	25–100	25–100
Clonidine	Catapres	0.1–.3	0.2–0.9

Figure 16-C

Beta Blockers

Beta blockers are medications that act by blocking the effects of norepinephrine at the receptor. They are very effective at reducing the peripheral manifestations of anxiety (increased heart rate, sweating, tremor), but are not very effective at blocking the internal experience of anxiety. They are used very effectively for the treatment of performance anxiety, such as that caused by public speaking. The most commonly used beta blocker is propranolol (Inderal), but atenolol (Tenormin) is also used (see figure 16-C). Beta blockers can cause dizziness and lowered blood pressure (in fact, their main use is as antihypertensives) and can cause depression if used over a long period of time. They have been used with some benefit as adjunctive agents in the treatment of panic disorder. Beta blockers are not habit forming, but should be discontinued slowly to avoid rebound elevation of blood pressure.

Clonidine

Clonidine (Catapres) is an alpha-2 adrenergic agonist, which thereby functions as a presynaptic inhibitor of norepinephrine release. It is usually used to treat hypertension (like the beta blockers) but has been used to treat anxiety disorders with some success. It is also used to treat opiate withdrawal. A typical starting dose is 0.1 mg two to three times daily (see figure 16-C). It is also available as a transdermal patch.

Length of Treatment

Antianxiety medications, especially benzodiazepines, can provide relief of anxiety regardless of the cause: situational stress, hyperthyroidism, or manic excitement (see figure 16-D). Of course, it is crucial to recognize and treat the underlying disorder. The use of benzodiazepines should be avoided until other measures have been tried (such as psychotherapy, relaxation training) or if anxiety is severe.

Benzodiazepines are very safe and effective in the short-term treatment of anxiety. However, prolonged use (over six months) may lead to tolerance and dependence. There have been several waves of public alarm about the abuse potential of benzodiazepines. Over ten years ago, there was much concern about Valium abuse, as portrayed in the book *I'm Dancing As Fast As I Can* (Gordon 1990). More recently, there has been much concern about abuse of Xanax and memory impairment due to Halcion.

Indications for Antianxiety Agents

- Adjustment reaction
- Phobic disorders
- Panic disorders
- Generalized anxiety disorder
- Obsessive-compulsive disorder
- Post-traumatic stress disorder
- Psychophysiological disorders related to anxiety (somatization disorder)
- Other disorders with prominent anxiety or agitation

Figure 16-D

Because of the potential for dependence and abuse, it is best to try to use benzodiazepines only for short-term treatment. (One bad experience with someone who abuses these drugs is enough to make you vow to never prescribe them long-term again.) The problem lies in identifying beforehand that small percentage of people at high risk for abuse. A prior history of substance abuse is, of course, a good predictor, but is not always present. On the other hand, many people take moderate doses of benzodiazepines for years without escalation in dose or any deleterious side effects. And some patients with panic disorder or other anxiety disorders who do not tolerate or respond to other forms of treatment (such as antidepressants or buspirone) do well on long-term maintenance with benzodiazepines without abuse developing. However, long-term benzodiazepine treatment is presently, and probably will remain, controversial.

Benzodiazepine Withdrawal

Minor tranquilizers and sedative-hypnotics are widely used in general medical practice and psychiatry. Although the benzodiazepines as a class are much safer than earlier medications (there is less risk of dependency and abuse, and withdrawal symptoms are generally much less dangerous than with barbiturates), problems do exist when patients begin to reduce doses, especially if they discontinue rapidly or "cold turkey." Benzodiazepine withdrawal syndromes are encountered frequently. They cause considerable patient distress, can be dangerous at times, and are almost always avoidable if the clinician follows the discontinuation guidelines carefully.

When patients are treated daily for more than a few weeks, especially in a moderate to high doses, the nervous system adapts to the presence of the drugs (tolerance develops) such that any rapid drop in blood levels of the medication can precipitate a withdrawal syndrome. Symptoms of withdrawal include the following (Smith and Wesson 1983):

Mild to Moderate	Severe
Anxiety	Seizures
Restlessness	High fever
Insomnia	Psychosis
Nightmares	Death

Typically, antianxiety medications with short half-lives (see figure 16-A) are more likely to produce withdrawal symptoms (since the medications are more rapidly eliminated from the system). However, clearly, withdrawal can occur with *all* minor tranquilizers and sedative-hypnotics (with the exception of buspirone and possibly zolpidem, which are chemical compounds unrelated to the benzodiazepines).

Often anxiety symptoms occur after medications are discontinued. It is sometimes difficult to distinguish between anxiety symptoms attributed to withdrawal, per se, and a reemergence of the primary anxiety associated with the original anxiety disorder. One defining feature is that symptoms that continue longer than two weeks tend to indicate the persistence of the underlying disorder. In such cases, discontinuation is premature (since the underlying disorder has not yet resolved) and continued treatment is warranted. However, withdrawal symptoms may mimic the anxiety symptoms, especially in panic disorder.

When symptoms are determined to be withdrawal, the medication should be restarted or returned to the dosage level previously used for chronic treatment. Then a *very gradual* withdrawal regime can be initiated, a 5 to 10 percent reduction of the daily dosage per week. With the shorter half-life tranquilizers, often the pace of medication discontinuance must be even more gradual; that is a longer time must be allowed between progressive decreases in dose.

For reasons that are not well understood, many patients find that it is especially difficult to discontinue the very last dose, even if discontinuation has proceeded well up to that point. For example, many patients have problems discontinuing the final dose of alprazolam (for example, 0.25 mg twice a day). It is advisable to not rush this final stage of drug phase out. It may be wise to take an additional month or two to gradually discontinue the medication, or in some cases you may want to consider ongoing treatment with what amounts to microdoses of these medications. If there are no noticeable side effects, there are really no contraindications for prolonged treatment with very low doses of minor tranquilizers.

Finally, severe cases of drug dependence (high doses) are most safely detoxed in the hospital. Phenobarbital is the "gold standard" for severe withdrawal syndromes, but pentobarbital or carbamazepine may also be used.

Patient Education

Patients who have been prescribed antianxiety medications should be cautioned about the risk of dependence, the dangers of combining these drugs with alcohol (the story of Karen Ann Quinlan can be helpful in this regard), and the possible impairment of coordination (including driving a car). You may find it helpful to have an agreement with your client that they will use the medications only for a specific length of time, such as one month. Some patients are too quick to ask for antianxiety medications, and some are too reluctant. Both of these represent problems that need to be dealt with. For example, some patients have severe, disabling anxiety or insomnia and need to be encouraged to take antianxiety medications for a short period of time. They need to be reassured that they will not become addicted after a few days of treatment.

Similarly, often people taking buspirone need a lot of encouragement to keep taking the medication long enough to get benefit. This is especially the case for those looking for a "quick fix." Studies show that the benefits of buspirone are still increasing after three to six months of use.

Patients who have been on the medications for some time need to be advised against abrupt discontinuation, which can lead to a severe withdrawal syndrome and possible convulsions. A reduction in dose is likely to lead to a reemergence of the anxiety symptoms for which the person is being treated, such as panic attacks. If this is due only to drug withdrawal, the symptoms usually subside within two weeks. For this reason, as stated above, it is best to taper off benzodiazepine dosage very slowly after prolonged use.

17

Antipsychotic Medications

Antipsychotic medications have truly revolutionized the treatment of psychotic disorders. Their effectiveness is so vastly superior to previous treatments that they have ushered in a new era in the treatment of severe mental illnesses. Chlorpromazine (Thorazine) was first used in 1952 as a postoperative sedative. It was subsequently used as a sedative for psychiatric patients, and it was soon discovered that it had antipsychotic properties. Soon other "phenothiazines" were developed.

When these drugs were first used in clinical settings, the mechanism of action was unknown, although the medications were clearly quite successful in reducing psychotic symptoms. Later research determined that antipsychotic medications acted by producing a chemical blockade of dopamine D_2 postsynaptic receptors and that their clinical potency correlated with their degree of dopamine blockade. This lead to the dopamine hypothesis of schizophrenia (see chapter 9).

Other, chemically distinct dopamine blockers were then developed, such as thiothixene, haloperidol, loxapine, molindone, and pimozide. All of these antipsychotics are potent dopamine blockers and collectively were called neuroleptics because they inadvertently cause certain neurological side effects (discussed below). More recently, atypical antipsychotic medications have been developed (clozapine and risperidone), which are effective antipsychotics yet are weak dopamine blockers and cause minimal neurological side effects. This group is discussed separately below.

Standard Antipsychotics

The phenothiazines and similar antipsychotics can be divided into high-potency and low-potency groups (see figure 17-A). In addition, they can be ranked according to their tendency to produce extrapyramidal symptoms (EPS) versus sedation and anticholinergic side effects (see figure 17-B).

Dosages of Antipsychotic Medication			
Generic Name	**Brand Name**	**Dosage Range (mg/day)**	**Equivalence[a] (mg)**
Low Potency			
Chlorpromazine	Thorazine	50–1500	100
Thioridazine	Mellaril	150–800	100
Clozapine[c]	Clozaril	300–900	50
Mesoridazine	Serentil	50–500	50
High Potency			
Molindone	Moban	20–225	10
Perphenazine	Trilafon	8–60	10
Loxapine	Loxitane	50–250	10
Trifluoperazine	Stelazine	10–40	5
Fluphenazine	Prolixin[b]	3–45	2
Thiothixene	Navane	10–60	5
Haloperidol	Haldol[b]	2–40	2
Pimozide	Orap	1–10	2
Risperidone[c]	Risperdal	4–16	1–2
Antiparkinson/ Anticholinergic Drugs			
Trihexyphenidyl	Artane	5–15	
Benztropine mesylate	Cogentin	1–8	
Biperiden	Akineton	2–8	
Amantadine	Symmetrel	100–300	

[a] Dose required to achieve efficacy of 100 mg chlorpromazine.
[b] Available in time-release IM formulation.
[c] Atypical antipsychotic.

Figure 17-A

Side Effects of Antipsychotic Medications			
Medication	Sedation	Extrapyramidal[a]	Anticholergenic[b]
Chlorpromazine	High	++	++++
Thioridazine	High	+	+++++
Clozapine	High	0	+++++
Mesoridazine	High	+	+++++
Molindone	Low	+++	+++
Perphenazine	Moderate	+++	++
Loxapine	Low	+++	++
Trifluoperazine	Low	++++	++
Fluphenazine	Low	+++++	++
Thiothixene	Low	++++	++
Haloperidol	Low	+++++	+
Pimozide	Low	+++++	+
Risperidone	Low	+	+

[a] Acute: Parkinson's dystonias, akathisia. Does not reflect risk for tardive dyskinesia.
[b] All neuroleptics may cause tardive dyskinesia.

Figure 17-B

Side Effects and Their Management

All neuroleptics, to a greater or lesser degree, produce the following side effects, which can be classified into five groups.

Extrapyramidal

The neuroleptics produce extrapyramidal side effects due to the blocking of dopamine receptors. In addition to producing a reduction in positive psychotic symptoms by blocking dopamine in the mesolimbic region, they unfortunately produce extrapyramidal symptoms by dopamine blockade in the basal ganglia. There are three types of acute extrapyramidal symptoms: Parkinsonian side effects are those that resemble Parkinson's disease, with slowed movements, decreased facial expression, resting tremor, and a shuffling gait. Dystonic symptoms involve sustained muscle spasms, usually of the neck or shoulder (such as torticollis) and can be quite frightening and painful. Akathisia refers to an intense feeling of restlessness. At times this side effect can be confused with psychotic agitation and thus mistakenly result in the physician increasing the dose of medication which results in increased akathisia. Severe akathisia can be very uncomfortable and is associated with increased noncompliance and increased risk of suicide.

Anticholinergic

Antipsychotic medications block acetylcholine receptors and thereby affect the parasympathetic nervous system. This leads to dry membranes (especially mouth and eyes), blurred vision (especially near vision), intestinal slowing (constipation), difficulty urinating, sedation, and sexual dysfunction. These symptoms may be very mild or, depending on the type of medication, quite severe and disabling.

Antiadrenergic

Antipsychotic medications produce alpha-adrenergic blockade, which leads to orthostatic hypotension. This means that when the person stands up, blood pressure drops precipitously, leading to a transient lightheadedness and potentially a fall and injury.

Tardive dyskinesia

All of the above side effects appear within the first few hours or days of treatment or with increases in dose. In contrast, the tardive dyskinesias (disorders involving involuntary movements) appear late in the course of treatment or when the medication is reduced or discontinued. These movements usually improve slowly over time, but they may persist for years even after the medication is discontinued.

Atypical side effects

As with all medications, certain people may have allergic reactions to antipsychotic medications. Weight gain is a common side effect. Agranulocytosis, a very serious blood disorder, was reported in the past, but it now appears to have been caused by a contaminant in some drug preparations and has not been reported recently. Hepatitis, similarly, has not been reported recently. Since the antipsychotics lower the seizure threshold, they may lead to grand mal seizures. They also interfere with temperature regulation and may lead to hyperthermia, especially when the person exercises during warm weather. Antipsychotics raise prolactin levels and this may cause lactation. Neuroleptic malignant syndrome (NMS) is a rare, but potentially fatal reaction to antipsychotic medication. It is characterized by fever, confusion, and rigidity. If not recognized and treated promptly it can lead to irreversible coma and death.

Symptoms that require immediate medication reevaluation are these:

Side Effects Calling for Medication Reassessment

- Confusion
- Falls
- Inability to urinate
- Prolonged or severe constipation
- Rash
- High fever (may be due to agranulocytosis or NMS)
- Involuntary movements
- Jaundice (yellowish discoloration of skin, including eyes)
- Severe sedation
- Severe restlessness
- Muscle spasm (such as torticollis)

Management

Many of the side effects of antipsychotic medications can be managed so that they are less troublesome to patients. This ensures that patients are more willing to comply in taking them. Some side effects, such as sedation, can be managed by reducing the dose or by switching to a less sedating antipsychotic. (One should always use the lowest effective dose—although determining what dose that is, is not always easy.) Extrapyramidal side effects can be reduced by switching to a less potent (and more sedating) antipsychotic. Additionally, extrapyramidal side effects typically are managed by the addition of an antiparkinsonian drug (such as benztropine, trihexyphenidyl, or biperiden; see figure 17-A). However, these medications also have side effects: dry mouth, blurred vision, and constipation, but are usually fairly well tolerated. Akathisia may be treated with antiparkinsonian drugs, beta blockers (such as propranolol) or both. Usually by adjusting the dose, changing medications, and/or adding adjunctive medications (such as an antiparkinsonian) the side effects of the antipsychotic medications can be reduced to a tolerable level.

Atypical Antipsychotics

In contrast to the neuroleptics, the atypical antipsychotics (clozapine and risperidone) are weak dopamine and serotonin blockers. Clozapine is effective in treating both positive and negative symptoms of schizophrenia and often is effective where other antipsychotic medications have failed. As many as 40 percent of those who have failed to respond to haloperidol and chlorpromazine respond to clozapine.

To date, clozapine has a very low incidence of extrapyramidal side effects and very few reported cases of tardive dyskinesia. It is very sedating and has some anticholinergic and antiadrenergic side effects (see figure 17-B). Sedation is the most troublesome side effect. Clozapine also lowers the seizure threshold and can cause hepatitis. However, the most serious side effect is a severe blood disorder, aplastic anemia, which has caused several deaths in the United States. This side effect can usually be avoided by weekly monitoring of the white blood cell count; this testing is required of all people taking the medication. Clozapine can cost as much as $10,000 per year because of this need for weekly blood tests, although such a cost is minimal when compared to the cost of chronic institutionalization. There have also been a few sudden deaths associated with clozapine, presumably cardiac in nature.

The dose is usually begun at 25 to 50 mg per day and increased by 25 mg per day, as tolerated, up to a total daily dose of 400 to 600 mg (see figure 17-A). Above 600 mg the incidence of seizures becomes significant.

Another atypical antipsychotic medication, risperidone, has recently been put on the market. It shares some features with clozapine, including lower incidence of EPS and greater efficacy in the treatment of negative symptoms compared to typical antipsychotics. However, notably, it does not appear to have the risk of lowered white blood counts and may be a very promising alternative to clozapine.

Choice of Medication

The antipsychotic medications tend to be effective in the treatment of psychotic symptoms, regardless of the disorder. They can be effective in substance-induced delusional disorders, delirium, schizophrenia, mania, delusional disorder, and so on. Standard antipsychotics tend to be much more effective for positive symptoms but do little to improve negative symptoms. The newer, atypical antipsychotics are more effective for negative symptoms although clearly not a panacea since they are successful in only about 30 percent of cases.

The choice of medication is generally based on three factors:

- If an antipsychotic medication has been used with success in the past, generally the same medication is again prescribed.

- The patient's motor state is important to consider. Typically, very agitated patients may be given a more sedating (low-potency) medication, whereas markedly regressed or withdrawn patients will be given a less sedating (high-potency) drug.

- The side effect profile of the drug chosen must be considered in relation to the individual patient (see figure 17-C). For example, in the elderly, drugs high in anticholinergic side effects are likely to increase confusion and memory problems, thus high-potency drugs are often used, such as haloperidol or perphenazine.

Individual differences in drug metabolism vary considerably, the dosage ranges are quite broad, and thus it is always difficult to know what dose will be required. People are usually started on a low dose and gradually titrated upward depending on clinical response and side effects. In the past, the use of high doses of antipsychotic medications, referred to as *rapid neuroleptization*, was popular. However, more recent studies have shown that moderate doses will produce the same eventual outcome (after ten days) with fewer side effects.

Length of Treatment

All psychotic symptoms do not respond in the same time frame when treated with antipsychotic medications. Typically, severe restlessness, agitation, and marked confusion may subside after a few hours or a few days of treatment. However, longer periods of treatment are generally necessary to resolve symptoms such as delusions, hallucinations, and thought disorder. Some patients may show improvement in these symptoms within a week or two, but in some chronic schizophrenics, many weeks of treatment may be required to gradually reduce these positive symptoms.

The length of treatment also depends on the type of disorder. In substance-induced psychoses, delirium, or brief reactive psychosis, the medication usually can be discontinued after the acute phase. In schizophreniform disorder and atypical psychosis, it is often necessary to continue the medication for six months in order to avoid relapse. As mentioned previously, many studies have shown that discontinuation of medication in schizophrenia is associated with higher relapse rates. The

---

Special Considerations in Choosing an Antipsychotic

Patient Type	Medication Choice
Child	Low dose
Elderly	High-potency, low dose
Anxious or agitated	Low-potency
Bipolar, manic	Low-potency[a]

[a] Use caution when combining with lithium (may produce encephalopathy).

Figure 17-C

general rule is to continue treating schizophrenics for at least one year following the remission of psychotic symptoms to prevent relapse. However, because of the risk of tardive dyskinesia, this judgment must be based on the patient's prior history and ongoing assessment of emerging side effects. Abnormal movements, which may signal the emergence of TD, should be checked for at least every six months, for example, by using the AIMS scale (see figure 17-D).

Patient Education

Psychotic disorders are always accompanied by significant functional impairment and great personal suffering. A very common problem, especially with schizophrenia, is relapse. Most often, relapse can be traced to noncompliance with the medication regime. Thus patient education becomes a very important part of treatment. Education involves helping patients to recognize prodromal symptoms of their illness (which may necessitate a dosage increase). Often it is helpful to discuss the prodromal period prior to a psychotic episode in detail to emphasize the particular symptoms that may serve as warning signs for that person. It is also vital that both patients and their families be educated about the effects and side effects of antipsychotic medications—particularly tardive dyskinesia—so that side effects can be properly managed. They should be reassured that most side effects can be reduced to tolerable levels.

Helping patients understand the reasons for taking the medication and the need to manage side effects is an important part of ensuring compliance. Education of the patient's spouse and family is also very important in this regard. Often family members are the first to notice a change in the patient's behavior necessitating a

---

AIMS
(Abnormal Involuntary Movement Scale)

Rate the presence of involuntary movements in the following areas according to severity: 1=none, 2=minimal, 3=mild, 4=moderate, 5=severe.

Muscles of facial expression	1 2 3 4 5
Lips and perioral area	1 2 3 4 5
Jaw	1 2 3 4 5
Tongue	1 2 3 4 5
Upper extremities	1 2 3 4 5
Lower extremities	1 2 3 4 5
Trunk	1 2 3 4 5
Overall severity of abnormal movements	1 2 3 4 5
Incapacitation due to abnormal movements	1 2 3 4 5
Distress due to abnormal movements	1 2 3 4 5
Problems with teeth or dentures	Yes/No
Usually wears dentures	Yes/No

Source: U.S. Department of Health, Education, and Welfare

Figure 17-D

medication adjustment. The patient's physician and psychotherapist play a crucial role in helping to educate the patient and in detecting early symptoms of relapse.

Psychotherapeutic Issues

Several issues are important in doing psychotherapy with someone with schizophrenia, where medication compliance is often an issue and where medication noncompliance is usually, eventually, associated with relapse. One goal is to recognize and take measures to minimize side effects. Several studies have shown that akinesia and akathisia are associated with medication noncompliance. Another issue is making the schizophrenic symptoms ego-dystonic to the patient. This may be a long process, involving repeatedly pointing out the ways in which the symptoms are dysfunctional in the patient's life.

Medication may be seen by the patient as intrusive and controlling or, alternatively, as comforting—a transitional, object-like extension of the therapist. Patients will be prone to interpret the medication in psychotic ways, especially when they are more symptomatic (and more in need of medication). When compliance remains a significant problem, consideration may be given to using one of the long-acting injectable forms of the antipsychotics (haloperidol decanoate or fluphenazine decanoate).

18

Red Flags:
When to Reevaluate

Previous chapters have discussed the diagnostic phase of treatment, in which the clinician makes initial decisions regarding possible referral for medication treatment. We have also outlined basic treatment strategies and medication doses. The non-medical therapist is crucially involved in monitoring patient response to medications: noting signs of symptomatic improvement, the emergence of adverse effects, and, at times, exacerbation of symptoms. Knowing what to look for and when to direct the patient back to the prescribing physician is an important task. In this chapter, we will address six important conditions or circumstances in which a re-referral is indicated: failure to respond, need for dosage adjustment, unexplained relapse, the onset of new medical conditions, side effect problems, and discontinuation of medication treatment.

Failure to Respond

As noted in earlier chapters, a positive medication response is rarely immediate. Most psychotropic medications require a number of days or weeks to reach adequate blood levels and produce physiologic changes that yield symptomatic improvement. Also, there exists tremendous variability from patient to patient regarding absorption and metabolism of medications, which affects the ultimate response time. Initial doses often must be raised gradually, as tolerance for side effects is achieved and blood levels of the medication approach therapeutic levels.

Critical to appropriate treatment is conducting an *adequate trial*. Adequate trials must assume that the correct diagnosis has been made and the patient has actually taken the medication as prescribed. Beyond this, the two most important variables to consider are dosage and length of treatment. A general rule with all psychotropics is to use the lowest dose that is effective, although at the same time not to under-treat. The clinician must be willing to increase doses in order to achieve meaningful results, while continuously monitoring for the emergence of side effects.

Generally, if patients have been treated with moderate to high doses of psy-chotropic medications (or at adequate blood levels) for four or five weeks without noticeable improvement, a re-referral should be made for dosage increase, augmenta-tion, perhaps a change to another class of medication. It is not unusual to encounter patients who have been treated for months (or even years!) on a particular drug or dose without symptomatic improvement. This is not appropriate. Any condition that warrants medication treatment is undoubtedly causing considerable suffering. There is no justifiable reason to mistreat or undertreat for a long period of time without carefully reevaluating the current treatment and making necessary adjustments.

Need for Dosage Adjustment

In addition to patients' failure to respond, therapists commonly encounter situations in which the patient has shown a positive response, but the symptomatic improve-ment is only partial. Many patients who show partial response can experience en-hanced improvement when doses are increased or medications are augmented. In such cases of partial response, a re-referral is warranted.

Unexplained Relapse

Sometimes a patient who has responded well to psychotropic medication treatment, will at some point experience emergence of symptoms—even when medications are continued. When this occurs, the clinician should consider the following common reasons:

- Failure to comply with treatment; for example, the patient has not been tak-ing medication as prescribed.

- The patient has started to drink alcohol excessively, which may exacerbate depression or anxiety symptoms and may also interfere with metabolism of the psychotropic medication. Other substance abuse may account for in-creased symptomatology.

- The patient has experienced a significant increase in psychosocial stressors.

- A medical condition has developed that may contribute to the development of psychiatric symptoms, such as thyroid disease.

- "Breakthrough symptoms": at times the underlying neurochemical disorder or metabolic activity of the individual undergoes a change that results in a reemergence of symptoms. In many cases of breakthrough symptoms, a dos-age adjustment (usually an increase in dose) may be successful.

- Tolerance to the drug can develop. This is uncommon; however, there is increasing evidence that some medications work well in early stages of some biologically based mental illnesses but are not as successful in later phases of the illness. For example, lithium is very effective in early episodes of bi-polar disorder but is less effective after a number of episodes. This probably does not represent true "tolerance" but rather a change in the underlying pathophysiology or neurochemical substrate.

Onset of New Medical Conditions

A patient may initially be able to tolerate and safely take psychotropic medications; however, the onset of certain physical conditions can change this, necessitating a re-referral. Such conditions include pregnancy, epilepsy, certain types of glaucoma and physiological changes associated with aging and kidney disease. Another time to re-evaluate medications is when the patient has an upcoming surgery, since psycho-tropics can interact with anesthetics administered before or during surgery or could also inhibit the healing process. Likewise, new prescription and over-the-counter medications added to cope with coexisting medical problems can cause drug inter-action problems (see appendix C). This is frequently seen in elderly patients, who often have a host of medical problems and take many medications.

Side Effect Problems

All psychotropic medications have side effects to a greater or lesser degree. Some side effects are minor, benign, and transient. Others are quite unpleasant and at times dangerous. Summarized in figure 18-A are the most common side effects as-sociated with the various classes of psychotropic medications. These are classified into three groups:

- Minor or benign: Many of these side effects diminish or disappear with con-tinued treatment as tolerance develops.

- Troublesome side effects: These can cause moderate levels of discomfort and may result in poor compliance.

- Potentially serious side effects: These may cause excessive discomfort and can actually be dangerous.

A re-referral is warranted in cases where side effects are troublesome or potentially serious or when clinical signs of drug toxicity appear (see figure 18-B).

When It Is Time to Discontinue

Once a patient has fully recovered, the question of when to stop medication arises. Often, even if the patient is asymptomatic, an abrupt discontinuation of medications can result in either relapse or withdrawal symptoms. The matter of when to stop is highly individual and depends heavily on three factors:

- The patient's history of previous episodes

- Your assessment of the patient's vulnerability to relapse

Side Effects of Psychotropic Medications

Medication Class	Mild or Benign	Troublesome	Potentially Serious
Antidepressants			
Tricyclics	Dry mouth Constipation Nasal congestion Mild sedation	Oversedation Sexual dysfunction Weight gain Hypotension Tremor Blurred vision Rash Uninary retention	Dizziness or falls, especially in the elderly Seizures Photosensitivity Cardiac arrhythmias Mania or hypomania Glaucoma Urinary retention Low white blood cell count Fever Sudden high fever with jaundice Priapism High white blood cell count Swollen lymph nodes Respiratory distress
SSRIs	Sweating Nausea or gas Diarrhea Constipation Dry mouth Sedation	Headache Anxiety Insomnia Weight loss Rash Sexual dysfunction	
MAOIs	Headaches Dizziness Dry mouth Constipation Hallucinations Nausea Diarrhea	Increased heart rate Blurred vision Weight gain Anxiety	Low blood pressure Falls Muscle spasms Hallucinations Hypertensive crisis

Figure 18-A

Side Effects of Psychotropic Medications
(continued)

Medication Class	Mild or Benign	Troublesome	Potentially Serious

Antipsychotics	Mild sedation
	Tremor
	Dry mouth
	Blurred vision
	Increased
	  perspiration
	Constipation
	Nasal congestion
		Rigidity
		Sexual dysfunction
		Oversedation
		Low blood
		pressure
		Extrapyramidal
		  symptoms
		Breast enlargement
			Urinary retention
			High blood pressure
			Severe rigidity,
			  especially with
			  fever, jaundice
			Abnormal movements
			Falls
			Confusion
			Liver toxicity
			Cardiac arrhythmia
			Photosensitivity

Mood Stabilizers			
Lithium	Nausea Tremor Weight gain	Memory problems Sedation Muscle weakness Vomiting Diarrhea	Oversedation Confusion Incoordination
Anticonvulsants	Sedation Nausea Vomiting Headache Tremor	Muscle twitching Rash Blurred vision Dizziness Weight changes	Confusion Urinary retention Bone marrow depression
Antianxiety Agents			

Benzodiazepines	Mild sedation
	Constipation
		Oversedation
		Confusion (especially
		  in the elderly)
		Parodoxical
		  stimulation
			Dizziness or falls
			Low blood pressure

Buspirone	Dizziness Nausea Headaches	Insomnia Nervousness Dysphoria	
Antihistamines	Drowsiness GI upset	Dry mouth Sexual dysfunction Low blood pressure	Difficulty breathing Urinary retention

Figure 18-A continued

Signs of Toxicity or Overdose

Antidepressants:[a]

- Oversedation
- Cardiac arrhythmia
- Falls
- Dilated pupils
- Confusion
- Psychosis
- Seizures
- Coma
- Agitation

Antipsychotics:

- Oversedation
- Hyperthermia
- Restlessness or agitation
- Seizures
- Rigidity
- Coma
- Falls
- Cardiac arrhythmia
- Confusion

Lithium:[a]

- Oversedation
- Confusion
- Incoordination
- Seizure
- Coma

Antianxiety Agents:

- Confusion
- Slurred speech
- Incoordination
- Falls
- Oversedation
- Coma

Anticonvulsants:

- Oversedation
- Confusion
- Incoordination
- Cardiac arrhythmia

[a] Severe overdoses oftentimes are fatal.

Figure 18-B

- The patient's feelings about discontinuing medications. Figure 18-C provides *very* general guidelines for length of treatment; each case must be evaluated individually.

It is important to note that people treated with benzodiazepines will develop a tolerance to the medication and if abruptly discontinued *will* have withdrawal symptoms—some of which can be serious. Slow tapering of doses is required and almost always can be safely accomplished (see "Benzodiazepine Withdrawal" in chapter 16). In general, it is wise to withdraw *all* psychotropic medications gradually, for example, antidepressants should be withdrawn gradually over a period of four to six weeks. A re-referral to the prescribing physician is warranted when, in your judgment, it is time to begin discontinuing treatment.

Finally from start to finish, ongoing collaboration and communication between psychotherapist and physician is important. Even at times when no problems exist, you may simply want to update the physician on the patient's progress.

Length of Continued Treatment After Patient Becomes Asymptomatic

Disorder	Time Frame
Major Depression	
First episode	6–12 months
Subsequent episodes	12–36 months or possibly indefinitely
Panic Disorder	
First episode	6 months
Subsequent episodes	12–24 months
Psychotic Disorder	
Brief psychotic episode (remitting quickly)	3 months
Schizophrenia and schizophreniform disorder	
First episode	12 months
Subsequent episodes	24 months to indefinite
Bipolar disorder	Generally requires ongoing prophylactic treatment
Obsessive-compulsive disorder	6 months[a]
Post-traumatic stress disorder	6 months[a]
Borderline personality disorder	6 months[a]

[a] The time frame for discontinuing has not been firmly established.

Figure 18-C

Epilogue

On the Horizon

These are exciting times in mental health and the neurosciences—new discoveries are being made each month. As this book goes to press, no less than two dozen new psychotropic medications are in the various phases of prerelease investigation and research. There is great promise for continued breakthroughs: new medications that may provide more safe, effective, and selective treatments for mental disorders.

There have been many advances in psychopharmacology over the past forty years and new treatments that have progressively resulted in decreases in emotional despair in many millions of people suffering from psychiatric disorders. Yet, in closing, we want to strongly underscore the importance of the human relationship in psychiatric treatment. Ultimately, loneliness, alienation, hopelessness, and demoralization are not to be cured with chemicals, but rather must be addressed in the arena of human contact and understanding. This is what psychotherapists do best. And, in collaboration with our medical psychiatric colleagues, we can make a real difference in the lives of our clients.

Appendix A

Pharmacokinetics

This appendix provides an expanded discussion of the pharmacokinetics of psycho-therapeutic agents presented in chapter 3. It is intended for therapists with a special interest in this area or for those who actively comanage medication-treated patients.

Absorption

Absorption is important not only as the initial step in the pharmacokinetic process, but also as a determinant of a crucial clinical parameter called *bioavailability*, defined as the amount of drug reaching systemic circulation (Winter 1988). The amount of the drug that is bioavailable is usually expressed as a percentage of the administered dose. Medications directly injected into a vein (intravenous) are nearly 100 percent bioavailable, whereas orally administered drugs produce variable patterns of bioavailability. For instance, demonstrated oral bioavailability for some antipsychotics and certain tricyclic antidepressants ranges from 30 to 60 percent (Hollister 1992). Bioavailability may be decreased by a physiological process called the *first-pass effect*, in which a significant amount of the drug is metabolized before reaching the bloodstream. Most tricyclics undergo extensive first-pass metabolism, contributing to their relatively low bioavailability.

The therapist may encounter the clinical ramifications of bioavailability in regard to the issue of generic medications. Bioavailability is the benchmark measurement for determining bioequivalence between brand name and generic products. With many medications, generic formulations meet bioavailability standards and can provide economical alternatives to brand name products. This can be an important issue for psychiatric patients with limited financial resources, who often will simply quit taking their medications because of the expense or will take them sporadically to "make them last longer."

However, absolute bioequivalence is not guaranteed for all generic products. Although the active ingredient may be quantitatively the same as in the brand name product, there may be differences in the manufacturing process or in the physical properties of the final preparation that can affect the rate and extent of drug absorption. From a practical standpoint, the patient may experience a variable or inadequate response from the generic product. Although this does not occur frequently, it is a factor to consider when a patient responds atypically to a drug—especially with medications that have a narrow therapeutic index, such as anticonvulsants and tricyclic antidepressants. Psychotropics with periodic reports of generic unequivalence include nortriptyline and carbamazepine. Advise patients taking these medications to avoid frequent switches from brand to generic preparations and changes between generic manufacturers.

Distribution

Distribution of a medication throughout the body is a two-phase process. Initially, distribution is preferential for organs with a rich supply of blood flow, such as the kidney, liver, heart, and brain. In the second phase, the drug moves into areas with less extensive circulation, such as muscle and fat tissue. In chapter 3 these latter areas of the body are referred to as reservoirs, sometimes called compartments. Eventually (usually within several minutes), equilibrium is established. At equilibrium the process of drug distribution is completed, and the flow of the drug between compartments is relatively stable. When, as for most drugs, equilibrium is reached rapidly, the body as a whole is considered to be a single compartment, and the distribution pattern is referred to as a "single-compartment model." In this case it is assumed that the drug is uniformly distributed throughout the body; in other words, the serum level of the drug is equal to the concentration in organs and tissues.

Some psychotherapeutic medications, however, demonstrate "two-compartment" distribution. In the two-compartment model equilibrium is reached more slowly because of significant movement of the drugs into muscle and fat cells. Also distribution is not uniform throughout the body. Depending on the physical or chemical properties of the drug, and upon the physiological state of the patient, the drug can be unequally distributed between organs and reservoirs. Ultimately, large concentrations of medications can accumulate in deep reservoir areas.

Due to individual physiologic differences, there can be wide variations in effective dosages of the same medication from patient to patient. Also, when a medication is stopped (by either therapeutic plan or noncompliance), complete elimination of the drug does not occur immediately, or even within known half-life parameters. This partially explains why recurrence of psychosis may not immediately appear in the noncompliant schizophrenic and why depressive symptoms reemerge weeks (or days) after an antidepressant is discontinued. (The therapist can help educate the patient as to the potential consequences of medication discontinuation.)

Circulating in the plasma are various proteins to which medications can attach. This process is called protein binding and provides another reservoir area for drugs. Only the unbound or "free" molecules of drug are able to cross cell membranes and reach an eventual site of action; thus a bound drug is inactive, whereas an unbound drug is active. Most psychotropic medications are bound extensively to serum proteins, usually albumin. Laboratory monitoring results typically indicate a total concentration that includes both bound and unbound drug.

Metabolism

Metabolism (biotransformation) of most drugs primarily occurs through the action of enzymes located predominately in the liver. These enzymes constitute the mixed function oxidase (MFO) or cytochrome P/450 system. The amount and activity of these enzymes are subject to change. For instance, enzyme activity and amount may be increased (called enzyme induction) by medications, such as carbamazepine (Tegretol) or by other conditions, such as smoking. Decreases in production or activity of enzymes (enzyme inhibition) can result from medications, such as cimetidine (Tagamet) or from diseases, such as cirrhosis or hepatitis. Additionally, there are individual variations in people's ability to metabolize medications. The by-products of metabolism are called metabolites. As discussed in chapter 3, metabolites may possess similar activity to the original drug (often called the parent compound), and these "active metabolites" may contribute to the intended effect of the medication. However, metabolites can also demonstrate different properties than the parent drug. An example is seen in the substantially longer half-lives that metabolites of some benzodiaze-pines exhibit compared to the parent compounds, which can potentially lead to drug accumulation.

Therapeutic Index

A critical pharmacokinetic parameter that directs safe and effective medication use is the *therapeutic index*. This parameter establishes a quantitative comparison between a drug's effective concentration and its toxic concentration. The closer these measurements are, the narrower the index, and therefore the more care that must be taken in prescribing. Lithium and anticonvulsants, for example, have narrow therapeutic indices.

Appendix B

Pharmacotherapy in Special Populations

Pregnancy

One of the most difficult dilemmas facing physicians is medication management in the psychiatric patient who is pregnant or considering pregnancy. Although therapists will not have to make ultimate prescribing decisions, they will undoubtedly remain involved in the patient's care. The information presented here summarizes general guidelines relevant to psychotropic medication use during pregnancy and nursing.[1]

It is important to remember that absolute data in this area is disturbingly incomplete. Experimental research obviously is limited by ethical restrictions. Animal studies are extensive but their results cannot be assumed to necessarily apply to humans. And, for infrequently prescribed medications, the available observational data are in some cases so limited that conclusions are impossible. Nevertheless, in some patients the risk of not medicating, especially in the presence of psychosis, mania,

---

1. Information from a variety of sources was compiled for this appendix: American Society of Hospital Pharmacists 1993; Brown and Bryant 1992; Ereshefsky and Richards 1992; Facts and Comparisons 1993; Jann 1992; Jinks and Fuerst 1992; Meyer 1992; Rubin 1992; Snodgrass 1992; Vestal, Montamat, and Nielson 1992.

and severe depression, clearly outweighs the potential hazards to mother and child. The risk factors are these:

Risk Factors Associated with Medications During Pregnancy

- Teratogenesis (malformation of fetus or fetal organs)
- Drug effects on the growing and developing fetus
- Drug effects on labor and delivery
- Residual drug effects on the newborn (neonatal)
- Behavioral teratogenesis (long-term effects on the child resulting from drug exposure in utero)
- Pregnancy-induced changes in drug actions
- Drug effects on the breastfed infant

Perhaps of most concern is the possibility of teratogenesis, with the risk being greatest during the period of organ formation (organogenesis) generally considered to be

---

Psychotropic Medication Guidelines for Pregnancy

Antidepressants:
- Fluoxetine and most tricyclics not associated with teratogenesis.
- Desipramine and nortriptyline are preferred. Can monitor serum levels.
- MAOIs and bupropion have not been studied extensively.
- Inconclusive data on miscarriage rate.
- Effects on neonate can include CNS depression, urinary retention.
- Present in breast milk.

Lithium:
- Established teratogen. First trimester exposure strongly associated with fetal cardiac anomaly.
- For fetal lithium exposure in first trimester, consider cardiac ultrasound to detect presence or absence of malformation.
- If lithium is necessary after first trimester, dosage adjustments are necessary due to pregnancy-induced kidney function changes. Frequent lab monitoring is also required.
- Reductions in lithium dose are required several weeks prior to delivery.
- Neonatal effects include impaired respiration, EKG and heart rate abnormalities, and renal impairment.
- Carbamazepine, clonazepam, and neuroleptics are possible alternatives to lithium.
- Significant concentrations in breast milk. Can cause decreased muscle tone, cyanosis, lethargy in infant. Nursing contraindicated.

Figure B-1

the first trimester. Avoiding medications as much as possible during this time can lower the risk of fetal malformation. However, since most drugs, with very few exceptions, cross the placenta, fetal medication exposure will continue throughout pregnancy. After the first trimester, safety concerns are related to effects on fetal growth and physiology, immediate and long-term effects on the child, and on breast feeding. Figure B-1 provides guidelines for psychotropic medication use in pregnancy and nursing.

Geriatric Patients

Increasingly, our society is composed of greater numbers of elderly individuals, defined as 65 and older. Currently, the elderly constitute nearly 20 percent of the population. Consequently, psychotherapists are faced with diagnostic and treatment dilemmas specific to this population. Presented here are patterns and risks of medication use in the elderly (figure B-2) and age-specific factors contributing to adverse effects (figure B-3). Also discussed are recommended adjustments for use of psychotropics in the geriatric patient.

Psychotropic Medication Guidelines for Pregnancy

(continued)

Antipsychotics:

- High-potency agents may be preferred over low-potency agents.
- Establish lowest effective dose possible.
- Potential short-term abnormal neonatal motor activity.
- Possible alternative to lithium in mania.
- Present in breast milk.

Anticonvulsants:

- Carbamazepine is possible lithium alternative. However, recent findings indicate that it is less safe than previously thought; probable teratogen.
- Valproic acid is established teratogen.
- Carbamazapine and valproic acid both found in breast milk.

Benzodiazepines:

- Some benzodiazepines have established role in fetal abnormalities. Avoid use in first trimester. May need to taper dose.
- Switch to clonazepam if benzodiazepines absolutely indicated.
- Switch to tricyclic antidepressant for panic disorder if continued medication is required.
- Neonatal CNS depression, drug accumulation, and withdrawal symptoms possible.
- Excreted in breast milk. Produces drowsiness, failure to thrive in infant.

Source: Cohen, Heller, and Rosenbaum 1989; Briggs 1992; Rubin 1992.

Figure B-1

Prescribing psychotropic medications in a population receiving numerous maintenance medications for medical conditions is inherently difficult. However, we present the following general recommendations to reduce the risk to this group.

Establish diagnosis and target symptoms

Neuroleptics are frequently prescribed for geriatric patients, especially in long-term care facilities. However, these drugs may not be prescribed for psychotic symptoms but may merely be intended to control agitation and anxiety. An alternative to neuroleptics and benzodiazepines is buspirone (BuSpar).

Obtain complete medication history

Elderly people are at higher risk for developing drug-induced psychiatric symptoms from other prescribed medications, such as depression secondary to cardiovascular drugs or delirium and confusion secondary to CNS medications. Frequently, yet another medication is prescribed as a result, without the real cause of symptoms (the medication) having been identified. Also, additive drug effects are common in the elderly. For example, it is important to evaluate the total number of anticholinergic drugs before adding another one, since geriatric patients are especially prone to "anticholinergic delirium." Lastly, multiple medications (such as antihypertensives and diuretics) can increase the possibility of psychotropic-related falls.

Understand age-specific pharmacology

Some benzodiazepines, such as diazepam (Valium), chlordiazepoxide (Librium), and flurazepam (Dalmane), accumulate to a greater degree than others. Benzodiazepines considered to be safer are oxazepam (Serax), lorazepam (Ativan), and temazepam (Restoril). Additionally, the elderly in general are more likely to experience oversedation from benzodiazepines.

The most consistently predicable age-related change in drug response results from the normal decrease in kidney function that accompanies aging. This phenomenon probably contributes to the greatest number of adverse drug reactions in the elderly (Jinks and Fuerst 1992). Safe use of lithium, therefore, becomes particularly difficult. Aggressive serum-level monitoring and assessment of renal function are imperative.

Central nervous system changes are common with aging, including decreased cerebral blood flow, decreased cholinergic function, increased monoamine oxidase ac-

---

Medication Use and Risks in Geriatric Patients

- 30 percent of all prescription drugs are taken by people over 65 years of age.

- 70 percent of older adults self-medicate with over-the-counter products without physician or pharmacist consultation.

- 50 percent of accidental drug-related deaths occur in geriatric patients.

- Adverse drug reactions occur at double the rate in geriatric patients than in other groups.

- Common adverse drug-related effects are hip fractures, cognitive impairment, and neuroleptic-induced parkinsonism.

Figure B-2

Contributing Factors to Adverse Drug Reactions in the Elderly

- Adverse drug reactions are proportional to the number of medications taken.

- Elderly patients often have multiple prescribers without consolidated records.

- Age-related factors increase the likelihood of adverse effects, such as the following:

    Impaired organ function, especially decreased liver metabolism leading to increased medication levels and effects

    Multiple disease states

    Exaggerated therapeutic response to medications

    Increased sensitivity to side effects

- Noncompliance in elderly is common (usually underdosing) and due to:

    Complicated directions

    Hearing and visual impairment

    Cognitive and memory deficits

    Child-resistant packaging

    Cost

Figure B-3

tivity, and some brain atrophy. The result of these alterations can include the appearance of behavioral changes in the elderly and unpredictable medication response. Therefore, it is advisable to avoid frequent medication changes and not to experiment with medications in the elderly.

Adjust dosage

All psychotropics prescribed to elderly patients should begin with small doses and be titrated slowly. In addition, maintenance doses may sometimes be 30 to 50 percent lower than in younger patients. The aging person may demonstrate increased receptor or organ sensitivity to medications and there is an age-associated decrease in albumin, resulting in more free (active) drug available.

In general, continuous attention should be paid to reducing the total number of drugs, eliminating duplicative agents, and simplifying the dosing schedule. Also, clearly instruct the patient and his or her spouse and family when medications are discontinued.

Use therapeutic monitoring

Liberally utilize laboratory monitoring capabilities.

Recognize and respond to side effects promptly

Psychotropic side effects that are more pronounced in the elderly are sedation, anticholinergic reactions, extrapyramidal symptoms, delirium, postural hypotension, cardiotoxicity, and cognitive impairments. Constipation is common and particularly troubling in the elderly. Therefore, add anticholinergic agents with caution, and recommend treatment at time of prescribing to prevent potentially serious gastrointestinal effects.

Children and Adolescents

Psychotherapeutic agents are routinely prescribed for children and adolescents. Figure B-4 presents a summary of prescribing recommendations for younger patients.

Patients with Unusual Medication Metabolism

The emerging fields of pharmacogenetics and pharmacoanthropology attempt to identify variations in drug response attributable to genetic or ethnic factors. The most commonly encountered alterations in drug reactions are exaggerated response, novel drug effects, and lack of effectiveness (Meyer 1992). The dynamics and kinetics of drugs in the body are determined by genetically mediated patterns of protein structures, receptor sensitivities, and enzyme activity. We present here established findings in this area, acknowledging that information is likely to expand rapidly in the future.

Differences in biotransformation capacities have been identified for at least two distinct groups: poor metabolizers and extensive metabolizers. Poor metabolizers demonstrate a deficiency in one or more pathways of the cytochrome P/450 enzyme system. Since the metabolism of antidepressants and neuroleptics depends on this system (see appendix A), poor metabolizers may be at risk for complications of therapy. For certain tricyclic antidepressants and neuroleptics, it has been established that these individuals will demonstrate increased serum levels and exaggerated medication response. Additionally, they will be more susceptible to side effects. Although data is limited on the SSRIs, similar patterns are evident.

Extensive metabolizers, conversely, may show lack of response even at relatively high doses. Also, the effect of interacting drugs may be more pronounced in extensive metabolizers. A noted clinical example is the metabolic inhibition of antipsychotics on TCAs, leading to elevated serum levels of the latter. It is estimated that 20 to 30 percent of all patients on antidepressants are either poor or extensive metabolizers (Meyer 1992). Therapeutic drug monitoring is an important tool in avoiding under- and overdosing in these populations.

Several other genetically determined metabolic pathways affect the rate and degree of metabolism of phenelzine (Nardil) and certain benzodiazepines. Unpredicted medication responses to these agents are potentially linked to altered metabolism.

Current research seeks to further define altered drug metabolizers along ethnic and racial lines. However, since some ethnic groups traditionally underutilize psychiatric services, complete data for these populations may be difficult to obtain.

Psychotropic Medication Guidelines
for Children and Adolescents

Antidepressants:

- Imipramine is the antidepressant most frequently prescribed for children and is the one most extensively studied in that population. Consider desipramine if anticholinergic side effects are to be avoided, for instance, in asthmatics.

- Dosage ranges are based on body weight: 1–5 mg/kg/day.

- EKG should be performed prior to treatment, when dosage reaches 3 mg/kg/day, and when heart rate is greater than 130 beats per minute. Repeat EKG is recommended when maintenance dose is reached, to minimize the possibility of toxicity.

- Do not exceed plasma concentration of 225 mg/ml (imipramine plus its desipramine metabolite) in children, due to increased risk of cardiovascular effects at higher serum levels.

- Preadolescent children demonstrate a shorter half-life of imipramine; therefore, several divided doses per day are required.

- More free drug is available in children, due to decreased protein binding and high proportion of lean body mass.

- Few established recommendations of SSRIs and MAOIs.

Lithium:

- Lithium is accepted as relatively safe in children and adolescents and is tolerated better by them than by adults.

- Starting dose for children is 30 mg/kg/day in divided doses. Starting dose for adolescents is the same as for adults: 900–1200 mg/day.

- Monitor children closely for dehydration, especially during periods of activity, seasonally hot temperatures, and illnesses associated with fever and fluid loss.

- Monitor for hypothyroidism to avoid growth retardation.

- Limited animal evidence demonstrates inhibited bone growth and lithium deposits in immature bones. Therefore, monitor calcium levels and maintain growth charts. For this reason, carbamazepine may be safer in children under age 12.

Anticonvulsants:

- Established anticonvulsant dosage and monitoring guidelines are generally followed for use in pediatric psychiatry.

- Monitor children for appearance of (or worsening of) cognitive and behavioral side effects associated with anticonvulsants. With caramazepine these can include insomnia, irritability, emotional lability, and impaired task performance. With valproic acid observe for excessive drowsiness and (minimal) effect on task performance.

Figure B-4

Psychotropic Medication Guidelines
for Children and Adolescents *(continued)*

Benzodiazepines:

- Although used medically (such as for seizures or during anesthesia) the benzodiazepines are not considered first-line agents for psychiatric symptoms in children.

- Childhood anxiety disorders may respond better to nonpharmacologic therapies. If medications are indicated, imipramine is more often recommended.

- If benzodiazepines are used in children, dosing should be designed to avoid excessive sedation relating to peak concentrations.

- Clonazepam reported to cause irritability, aggression, and antisocial features in children.

Antipsychotics:

- For many antipsychotics there are established dosing guidelines, based on body weight, for children aged 3 to 12 years. Adult dosages are usually applied to children over 12.

- Phenothiazines should be used cautiously in children with acute illnesses, such as chicken pox, measles, or GI or CNS infections, due to increased susceptiblilty to dystonia and akathisia.

- Neuroleptics may cause an allergic reaction, including breathing difficulties. Use cautiously in childhood asthma.

- Acute dystonic reactions occur more often in children and adolescents than in adults. For younger children, diphenhydramine (Benadryl) is a common treatment, although other anticholinergics may be used.

- Children, but not adolescents, demonstrate shorter half-lives with antipsychotics, and consequently may not be good candidates for once-a-day dosing.

Psychostimulants:

- Dosage guidelines based on body weight:

    Methylphenidate (Ritalin) 0.3–3 mg/kg/day

    Dextroamphetamine (Dexedrine) 0.5–2 mg/kg/day

    Pemoline (Cylert) 2.25 mg/kg/day

- Give with meals to minimize GI distress and appetite loss.

- Give doses early in the day to avoid insomnia.

- Growth suppression associated with dextroamphetamine and methylphenidate has not been clearly established; if it does occur it is not permanent.

Figure B-4

Appendix C

Psychotropic Drug Interactions

This appendix provides a quick reference guide to frequent and significant drug interactions between psychotropic medications.[1] These tables are not absolute. Interactive effects will vary from person to person. In some instances an individual may experience the full range of symptoms presented here, while others may demonstrate only one or two symptoms from a range of possible effects.

Also note that the potential for an interaction between drugs does not preclude their concurrent use. Certain combinations are routinely prescribed without problems in many patients (as with lithium and antipsychotics), whereas others are contraindicated due to the severity of the interaction (for example, MAOIs and SSRIs). *However, whenever psychiatric medications are coadministered, the additive potential of central nervous system depression and anticholinergic effects must be considered.*

---

1. Information from a variety of sources was compiled for this appendix: American Society of Hospital Pharmacists 1993; Facts and Comparisons 1993; Hansten and Horn 1993; Watsky and Salzman 1991.

Tricyclic Antidepressant (TCA) Interactions

Drug	Effect of Interaction
Cimetidine (Tagamet)	Increased TCA levels, enhanced TCA response, TCA toxicity
Fluoxetine (Prozac)	
Propoxyphene (Darvon, Darvocet)	
Anticonvulsants Carbamazepine (Tegretol) Phenytoin (Dilantin) Barbiturates (phenobarbital)	Decreased TCA levels, diminished TCA response
MAOIs—**contraindicated with TCA** especially with imipramine and clomipramine; trazodone may be used cautiously with MAOIs	Increased TCA levels; syndrome of excitation, very high temperature, mania, seizures, coma, **death**
Clonidine (Catapres) Guanethidine (Ismelin)	Decreased antihypertensive effect of clonidine and guanethidine
Quinidine	Increased TCA levels, TCA-induced cardiac conduction prolongation
Antipsychotics	Increased TCA levels
Lithium	May worsen lithium tremor, increased TCA effect

Selective Serotonin Re-uptake Inhibitor (SSRI) Interactions

Drug	Effect of Interaction
MAOIs—**contraindicated with SSRIs**	Serotonergic syndrome with symptoms of fever, tremor, muscular rigidity, seizure, coma, **death**
TCAs	Increased TCA levels (*may be significant, doubled or greater*), enhanced TCA response, TCA toxicity
Carbamazepine (Tegretol)	Increased carbamazepine levels
Lithium	Increased lithium levels, possible neurotoxicity (confusion, dizziness, tremor, muscle stiffness, incoordination)
L-Tryptophan	Headache, nausea, restlessness, agitation, sweating

Note: Certain interactions with the SSRIs are assumed to occur with all medications in this category. For instance, all SSRIs should be avioded with MAOIs. However, interactions involving metabolic pathways, such as with carbamazepine, may be more likely with one SSRI than with others, since not all SSRIs are metabolized identically. Also, due to the relatively recent introduction of the SSRIs, it is possible that other drug interactions will be identified as these agents gain wider use.

Monoamine Oxidase Inhibitor (MAOI) Interactions

Drug	Effect of Interaction
Amphetamines—**contraindicated with MAOIs** Methylphenidate (Ritalin)—**contraindicated with MAOIs**	Seriously elevated blood pressure (hypertensive crisis), elevated temperature, seizures, cerebral hemorrhage, **death**
Ephedrine[a]—**contraindicated with MAOIs** Pseudoephedrine[b]—**contraindicated with MAOIs** Phenylephrine[b]—**contraindicated with MAOIs** Phenylpropanolamine[c]—**contraindicated with MAOIs**	Seriously elevated blood pressure (hypertensive crisis), elevated temperature, seizures, cerebral hemorrhage, **death**
L-dopa—**contraindicated with MAOIs**	Seriously elevated blood pressure (hypertensive crisis), elevated temperature, seizures, cerebral hemorrhage, **death**
Buspirone (BuSpar)—**contraindicated with MAOIs**	Seriously elevated blood pressure (hypertensive crisis), elevated temperature, seizures, cerebral hemorrhage, **death**
Dextromethorphan[d]	Nausea, elevated temperature, low blood pressure, agitation, seizures, coma
Meperidine (Demerol)—**contraindicated with MAOIs**	Severe reactions with symptoms of hypertension, muscular rigidity, coma, **death**
TCAs (especially imipramine and clomipramine)—**contraindicated with MAOIs** (trazodone may be used cautiously with MAOIs)	Increased TCA levels; syndrome of excitation, very high temperature, mania, seizures, coma, **death**
Serotonin specific reuptake inhibitors (SSRIs)—**contraindicated with MAOIs**	Serotonergic syndrome with symptoms of fever, tremor, muscular rigidity, seizure, coma, **death**
L-Tryptophan	Hyperthermia, confusion, disorientation, agitation

[a] Common ingredient in over-the-counter allergy/asthma products
[b] Common ingredient in over-the counter cold/allergy products
[c] Common ingredient in over-the-counter cold/allergy products and nonprescription diet aids
[d] Common ingredient in over-the-counter cough syrups

Lithium Interactions

Drug	Effect of Interaction
Diuretics, especially thiazides	Increased lithium levels, lithium toxicity
Nonsteroidal anti-inflammatory agents Ibuprofen (Motrin, Advil, Nuprin) Naproxen (Naprosyn) Indomethacin (Indocin) Piroxicam (Feldene)	Increased lithium levels, lithium toxicity
Angiotensin converting enzyme inhibitors Captopril (Capoten) Enalapril (Vasotec) Lisinopril (Zestril, Prinivil)	Increased lithium levels, lithium toxicity
Metronidazole (Flagyl)	Increased lithium levels, lithium toxicity
Calcium channel blockers Verapamil (Calan, Isoptin) Diltiazem (Cardizem)	Increased or decreased lithium levels, neurotoxicity (weakness, incoordination, muscle stiffness, abnormal movements, psychosis)
Antipsychotics	Neurotoxicity (delirium, seizures, encephalopathy) or increased extrapyramidal symptoms
Carbamazepine (Tegretol)	Neurotoxicity (*not* associated with increase in lithium level)
TCAs	Possible worsening of lithium tremor, increased TCA effect
SSRIs	Increased lithium levels, possible neurotoxicity (confusion, dizziness, tremor, muscle stiffness, incoordination)
Theophylline Caffeine	Decreased lithium levels
Sodium chloride (high doses) Sodium bicarbonate (high doses)	Decreased lithium levels

Antipsychotic Interactions

Drug	Effect of Interaction
Amphetamines	Increased psychosis

Anticonvulsants
   Carbamazepine (Tegretol)
   Phenobarbital
	Decreased antipsychotic levels, increased sedation

Meperidine (Demerol)	Hypotension, lethargy
L-dopa	Decreased effectiveness of L-dopa in parkinsonism
Isoniazid (INI I)	Liver toxicity, encephalitis
Anesthetics	Hypotension
Lithium	Neurotoxicity (delirium seizures, encephalopathy) or increased extrapyramidal symptoms
TCAs	Increased TCA levels
Beta blockers	Increased levels of both drugs, hypotension

Anticonvulsant (Carbamazepine (CBZ) and Valproic Acid (VA))

Drug	Effect of Interaction

Cimetidine (Tagamet)
Calcium channel blockers
   Verapamil (Calan, Isoptin)
   Diltiazem (Cardizem)
Fluoxetine (Prozac)
Propoxyphene (Darvon, Darvocet)
Erythromycin and related antibiotics
	Increased CBZ levels, CBZ toxicity (drowsiness, dizziness, nausea, vomiting, blurred vision, slurred speech, cardiac problems)

Other anticonvulsants
   Phenytoin (Dilantin)
   Phenobarbital
	Increased or decreased CBZ and VA levels, increased or decreased levels of other anticonvulsants

Aspirin	Increased VA levels
TCAs Anticoagulants Antipsychotics Theophylline Oral contraceptives Doxycycline	CBZ decreases serum levels, diminished effect of listed drugs
Lithium	Neurotoxicity with litihum and CBZ (*not* associated with increase in lithium level)

Benzodiazepine Interactions

Drug	Effect of Interaction
Disulfiram (Antabuse) Cimetidine (Tagamet) Isoniazid (INH) Oral contraceptives	Increased benzodiazepine levels
Alcohol, CNS depressants (narcotics, barbiturates)	Potentiate CNS depression
L-dopa	Decreased effectiveness of L-dopa in parkinsonism
Bupropion (Wellbutrin)	Abrupt benzodiazepine withdrawal increases seizure risk

Miscellaneous Drug Interactions

Interactive Combination	Effect of Interaction
Bupropion (Wellbutrin) and benzodiazepines	Abrupt benzodiazepine withdrawal increases seizure risk
Bupropion (Wellbutrin) and L-dopa	Excitability, restlessness, tremor, nausea, vomiting
Buspirone (BuSpar) and MAOIs—**contraindicated**	Seriously elevated blood pressure (hypertensive crisis), elevated temperature, seizures, cerebral hemorrage, **death**

Appendix D

Differentiating Psychotropic Side Effects from Psychiatric Symptoms

In this appendix we discuss a potentially problematic area: the identification of, and response to, psychotropic-induced side effects. The most obvious danger of failing to accurately differentiate medication side effects from a disease process is the possibility that one might increase the dose of the very medication responsible for the the side effects. Similarly, unwarranted diagnoses may be assigned or unnecessary medications added.

At times, making this distinction is nearly impossible. Not only is the clinician required to separate strikingly similar medication side effects and psychiatric symptomatology, but the patient may be only marginally able to give a useful subjective description.

Akathisia Versus Agitation Associated with Worsening Anxiety or Psychosis

Akathisia, the compulsion to be in motion, may present with a variety of associated symptoms. Patients often experience an inability to remain still, pace, tap their feet while sitting, and shift their weight while standing. Along a continuum, mild akathisia may appear as increasing or emerging anxiety, and when more severe, may be mistaken for worsening psychosis.

Akathisia secondary to neuroleptics is more common in younger patients or with high-potency agents. The onset of akathisia can follow a variable course, appearing either early in treatment or up to several months later. Especially if the patient is not receiving anticholinergics, the possibility of medication-induced akathisia should be considered before more neuroleptic is administered. If symptoms diminish in response to anticholinergics, it is probably akathisia. If symptoms resolve with additional neuroleptic, it is more likely disease exacerbation. In some patients, response to anticholingerics is inadequate, requiring adding, or changing to, a benzodiazepine or beta blocker. In these cases, the patient will usually report a "physical" restlessness as opposed to "emotional" anxiety or agitation.

Akathisia has also been reported with the SSRIs, especially fluoxetine, and with the tricyclic antidepressants. Failure to recognize antidepressant-induced akathisia may lead to unnecessary prescribing of antianxiety agents or neuroleptics.

Excessive Anticholinergic Effects Versus Psychosis

An acute onset of primary organic symptoms may signal anticholinergic delirium, with associated mental status changes of confusion, disorientation, and tactile or visual hallucinations. Physiologic indicators include dry mucous membranes, increased heart rate, and dilated pupils. Recovery usually occurs within several days following discontinuation of the suspected anticholinergic drug, but occasionally this syndrome may last up to two weeks. Elderly people are especially prone to anticholinergic overload.

Drug treatment of anticholinergic delirium is typically not recommended, although benzodiazepines can be used to treat severe agitation. Neuroleptics, with their anticholinergic properties, are relatively contraindicated.

Parkinsonian Side Effects Versus Depression

Neuroleptic-induced parkinsonian side effects are characterized by the triad of tremor, muscle stiffness, and slowness of motion. For the most part, these physical indicators are relatively easy to identify. The tremor, which is somewhat coarse and may include classic "pill-rolling," is worse at rest, and is distinguishable from the fine, intention tremor of lithium. Muscle stiffness or rigidity is notable for the increased resistance to passive movement ("cogwheeling").

The absence of movement (akinesia) does not occur as frequently as slowed movement (bradykinesia). Moderate to severe bradykinesia includes postural abnormalities of shuffling gait, stooped appearance, and feeling off balance. Drooling and slowed, nonexpressive speech are also common. It is the mildly bradykinetic patient, without noticeable tremor or rigidity, whose presentation can mimic a depressive mood disorder. Overall, the slowed motion, lack of facial expression, apathy, and social withdrawal present markedly similar to depression. A careful evaluation should be made to determine the presence of associated parkinsonian characteristics before revising a diagnosis or initiating an antidepressant.

Acute Dystonia Versus Tardive Dyskinesia

Dystonic reactions occur within hours or days of initiating treatment with (or increasing the dose of) a neuroleptic. Tardive dyskinesia (TD) presents with a more insidious onset and is associated with long-term neuroleptic treatment. Figure D-1 summarizes the characteristics of acute dystonia and TD.

Not only is there no effective treatment for TD, but administration of anticholinergics is likely to worsen the symptoms. Therefore, the differential diagnosis of these two syndromes is critically important.

Acute Dystonia Versus Tardive Dyskinesia

Acute Dystonia

Fixed upward gaze (oculogyric crisis)

Neck twisting (torticollis)

Arching of the head backward (opisthotonos)

Clenched jaw or "lockjaw" (trismus)

Facial grimacing due to involuntary muscle contraction

Difficulty swallowing

Difficulty breathing (larynogospasm)

Tardive Dyskinesia

Abnormal, involuntary, rhythmic movements of the mouth, tongue, and lips, including protruding tongue, worm-like tongue movements, mouth puckering, lip smacking, and chewing motions

Irregular, purposeless, involuntary quick movements of the extremities, flailing or jerky in appearance

Continuous, writhing movements of extremities, including trunk or pelvis

---

Figure D-1

Antidepressant Toxicity Versus Worsening or Reemerging Depression

Symptoms of depression that reappear, or are slow to resolve with antidepressant treatment, may be explained by several factors, including noncompliance and poor therapeutic response requiring a medication change. Consideration should also be given to medication-related CNS toxicity. The most obvious of these symptoms that are also diagnostic of depression are irritability, confusion, memory impairment, anxiety, agitation, and lethargy. In determining a differential diagnosis, the clinician can assess for the physiologic symptoms of antidepressant toxicity (as described in chapters 14 and 18) and utilize laboratory monitoring for antidepressant blood levels.

Appendix E

Neurocognitive Mental Status Exam

Figure E-1 is a short exam that can be administered to patients as an aid in making a diagnosis. Notes on each question appear below. For a more comprehensive review of a neurologically based mental status exam, the reader is referred to an excellent text: *The Mental Status Examination in Neurology* (Strub and Black 1985).

Brief Neurocognitive Mental Status Exam

Name_____Age_____Date_____

Level of education_____Occupation_____

Onset of symptoms_____

Medications_____

_____

_____

1. Behavioral observations

    a. Level of awakeness/alertness_____

    b. Signs of impaired attention or distractibility_____

    c. Quality of speech_____

    d. Gait_____

2. Orientation: Time_____Place_____Person_____

3. Recent memory (three-item recall with five-minute delay)

    Trial A: House, Orange, Robert_____

    Trial B: Petunia, Buick, Wind_____

4. Calculations: 100 – 93 – 86 – 79 – 72 – 65 – 58 – 51_____

5. Reproduction of cross_____cube_____

6. Thinking/Speech: Coherent?_____Relevant?_____

Figure E-1

Notes on the Use of the Brief Neurocognitive Mental Status Exam

1. *Behavioral observations*

   a. Look for signs of drowsiness or fluctuating degrees of alertness.

   b. This may be formally tested by administering a digit span test or by careful observation during the interview.

   c. Make note of slurred speech or word-finding problems.

   d. Watch for unsteady gait and poor gross motor coordination.

2. *Orientation*—ask: "What is the date (month, day, year) and what time of day is it now?" "Can you tell me where you are right now? Please be specific." Ask the patient to identify relatives that have accompanied him or her.

3. *Recent memory*—present three items and ask for immediate recall. Then after a period of five minutes ask the patient to again recall the three items. Most normal adults should be able to recall three items. Inability to do so may suggest recent memory problems. A second trial may be conducted later in the interview.

4. *Calculations*—ask the patient to begin with the number 100 and subtract 7 from this number, then subtract 7 again, and so forth. This test provides a rough measure of concentration.

5. *Reproduction of cross and cube*—present stimulus illustrations shown below. You can copy them onto a 3-by-5-inch, unlined, white index card. Allow the patient to copy the designs one at a time onto a blank sheet of paper. Drawing performance can be compared to samples (see figure E-2) to derive rough estimates of the patient's constructional ability.

Cross   **Cube**

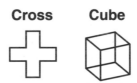

6. *Thinking/Speech*—note the presence of incoherent or irrelevant speech.

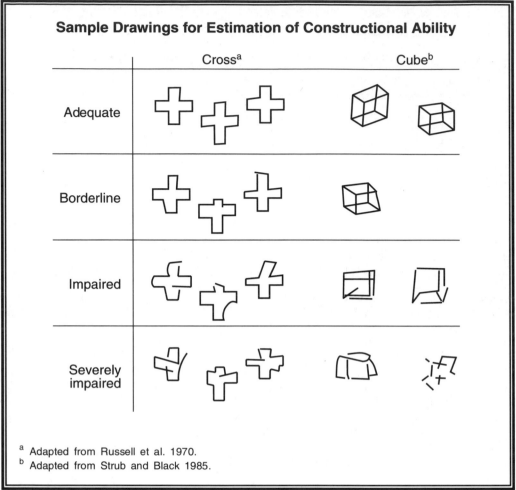

Sample Drawings for Estimation of Constructional Ability

	Cross[a]	Cube[b]
Adequate		
Borderline		
Impaired		
Severely impaired		

[a] Adapted from Russell et al. 1970.
[b] Adapted from Strub and Black 1985.

Figure E-2

Appendix F

Trade Versus Generic Drug Names: A Quick Reference

The following tables will enable you to quickly find the corresponding generic or trade name of a medication when you know only one of its names

Trade to Generic

Trade Name	Generic Name	Trade Name	Generic Name
Akineton	Biperiden	Mellaril	Thioridazine
Ambien	Zolpidem	Moban	Molindone
Anafranil	Clomipramine	Nardil	Phenelzine
Artane	Trihexyphenidyl	Navane	Thiothixene
Asendin	Amoxapine	Norpramin	Desipramine
Atarax	Hydroxyzine HCl	Orap	Pimozide
Ativan	Lorazepam	Pamelor	Nortriptyline
Aventyl	Nortriptyline	Parnate	Tranylcypromine
Benadryl	Diphenhydramine	Paxil	Paroxetine
BuSpar	Buspirone	Paxipam	Halazepam
Catapres	Clonidine	Permitil	Fluphenazine
Centrax	Prazepam	Prolixin	Fluphenazine
Clozaril	Clozapine	ProSom	Estazolam
Cogentin	Benztropine	Prozac	Fluoxetine
Cylert	Pemoline	Restoril	Temazepam
Dalmane	Flurazepam	Risperdal	Risperidone
Depakene	Valproic acid	Ritalin	Methylphenidate
Depakote	Valproic acid	Serax	Oxazepam
Desyrel	Trazodone	Serentil	Mesoridazine
Dexedrine	Dextroampheta-mine	Sinequan	Doxepin
		Stelazine	Trifluoperazine
Doral	Quazepam	Surmontil	Trimipramine
Effexor	Venlafaxine	Symmetrel	Amantadine
Elavil	Amitriptyline	Taractan	Chlorprothixene
Eldepryl	Selegiline (deprenyl)	Tegretol	Carbamazepine
Eskalith	Lithium carbonate	Tenormin	Atenolol
Eskalith CR	Lithium carbonate controlled release	Thorazine	Chlorpromazine
		Tindal	Acetophenazine
Halcion	Triazolam	Tofranil	Imipramine
Haldol	Haloperidol	Tranxene	Clorazepate
Inderal	Propranolol	Trilafon	Perphenazine
Klonopin	Clonazepam	Valium	Diazepam
Librium	Chlordiazepoxide	Versed	Midazolam
Lithonate	Lithium carbonate	Vistaril	Hydroxyzine pamoate
Lithotabs	Lithium carbonate	Vivactil	Protriptyline
Loxitane	Loxapine	Wellbutrin	Bupropion
Ludiomil	Maprotiline	Xanax	Alprazolam
Marplan	Isocarboxazid	Zoloft	Sertraline

Generic to Trade

Generic Name	Trade Name
Acetophenazine	Tindal
Alprazolam	Xanax
Amantadine	Symmetrel
Amitriptyline	Elavil
Amoxapine	Asendin
Atenolol	Tenormin
Benztropine	Cogentin
Biperiden	Akineton
Bupropion	Wellbutrin
Buspirone	BuSpar
Carbamazepine	Tegretol
Chlordiazepoxide	Librium
Chlorpromazine	Thorazine
Chlorprothixene	Taractan
Clomipramine	Anafranil
Clonazepam	Klonopin
Clonidine	Catapres
Clorazepate	Tranxene
Clozapine	Clozaril
Desipramine	Norpramin
Dextroamphetamine	Dexedrine
Diazepam	Valium
Diphenhydramine	Benadryl
Doxepin	Sinequan
Estazolam	ProSom
Fluoxetine	Prozac
Fluphenazine	Prolixin, Permitil
Flurazepam	Dalmane
Halazepam	Paxipam
Haloperidol	Haldol
Hydroxyzine HCl	Atarax
Hydroxyzine pamoate	Vistaril
Imipramine	Tofranil
Isocarboxazid	Marplan
Lithium carbonate	Lithotabs, Lithonate, Eskalith

Generic Name	Trade Name
Lithium carbonate, long acting	Eskalith CR
Lorazepam	Ativan
Loxapine	Loxitane
Maprotiline	Ludiomil
Mesoridazine	Serentil
Methylphenidate	Ritalin
Midazolam	Versed
Molindone	Moban
Nortriptyline	Pamelor, Aventyl
Oxazepam	Serax
Paroxetine	Paxil
Pemoline	Cylert
Perphenazine	Trilafon
Phenelzine	Nardil
Pimozide	Orap
Prazepam	Centrax
Propranolol	Inderal
Protriptyline	Vivactil
Quazepam	Doral
Risperidone	Risperdal
Selegeline (deprenyl)	Eldepryl
Sertraline	Zoloft
Temazepam	Restoril
Thioridazine	Mellaril
Thiothixene	Navane
Tranylcypromine	Parnate
Trazodone	Desyrel
Triazolam	Halcion
Trifluoperazine	Stelazine
Trihexyphenidyl	Artane
Trimipramine	Surmontil
Valproic acid	Depakote, Depakene
Venlafaxine	Effexor
Zolpidem	Ambien

Appendix G

Books for Patients About Medication Treatment

Depression

You Can Beat Depression: A Guide To Recovery, by J. Preston. San Luis Obispo, Calif.: Impact Publishers, 1991.

Feeling Good, by D. Burns. New York: New American Library, 1980.

Depression and Its Treatment, by J. Greist and J. Jefferson. New York: Warner Books, 1984.

The Depression Workbook, by Mary Ellen Copeland. Oakland, Calif.: New Harbinger Publications, 1992.

Bipolar Disorder

Mood Swings, by R. Fieve. Toronto: Bantum Books, 1975.

Lithium and Manic Depression: A Guide. Madison, Wis.: Lithium Information Center, University of Wisconsin, 1989.

Anxiety

The Anxiety Disease, by D. Sheehan. Toronto: Bantam Books, 1983.

Anxiety and Its Treatment, by J. Greist, J. Jefferson, and I. Marks. New York: Warner Books, 1986.

The Anxiety and Phobia Workbook, by Edmund Bourne. Oakland, Calif: New Harbinger Publications, 1990.

Psychosis

Surviving Schizophrenia: A Family Manual, by E. F. Torrrey. New York: Harper and Row, 1983.

Alzheimer's Disease

The 36-Hour Day: by N. L. Mace and P. V. Rabins. New York: Warner Books, 1981.

Obsessive-Compulsive Disorder

The Boy Who Couldn't Stop Washing, by J. Rapoport. New York: Signet Books, 1989.

When Once Is Not Enough, by Gail Steketee and Kerrin White. Oakland, Calif.; New Harbinger Publications, 1990.

Attention Deficit Disorder

The A.D.D. Hyperactivity Workbook, by H. C. Parker. Manassus, Va.: Impact Publications, 1988.

Borderline Personality Disorder

I Hate You—Don't Leave Me, by J. Kreisman and H. Kraus. Los Angeles: Price Stern Publishers, 1989.

Medications and Psychotherapy

Growing Beyond Emotional Pain, by J. Preston. San Luis Obispo, Calif.: Impact Publishers, 1993.

References

Agras, S. 1985. *Panic: Facing fears, phobias, and anxiety.* New York: W. H. Freeman.

Akiskal, H. S., and R. E. Weise. 1992. The clinical spectrum of so-called "minor" depressions. *American Journal of Psychotherapy.* 46:9–22.

American Society of Hospital Pharmacists. 1993. American hospital formulary service drug information. Bethesda, MD: American Society of Hospital Pharmacists.

Avis, H. 1990. *Drugs and life.* Dubuque, Iowa: W. C. Brown and Benchmark.

Ballenger, J. C., and R. M. Post. 1980. Carbamazepine in manic-depressive illness: A new treatment. *American Journal of Psychiatry.* 137:782–90.

Baron, M., N. Risch, R. Hamburger, B. Mandel, S. Kushner, M. Newman, D. Drumer, and R. Belmaker. 1987. Genetic linkage between X chromosome markers and bipolar affective illness. *Nature.* 326:289–92.

Baxter, L. R. 1991. PET studies of cerebral function in major depression and obsessive-compulsive disorder: The emerging profrontal cortex consensus. *Annals of Clinical Psychiatry* 3:103–09.

Baxter, L. R., J. M. Schwartz, K. S. Bergman, M. P. Szuba, B. H. Guze, J. C. Marriotta, A. Alazvaki, C. E. Selin, H. K. Feung, P. Munford, and M. E. Phelps. 1992. Caudate glucose metabolic rate changes with both drug and behavior therapy for obsessive-compulsive disorder. *Archives of General Psychiatry* 49:681–89.

Beardsley, R. S., G. J. Gardocki, D. B. Larsen, and J. Hidalgo. 1988. Prescribing of psychotropic medication by primary care physicians and psychiatrists. *Archives of General Psychiatry* 45:1117–19.

Beasley, C. M., and B. E. Dornseif. 1991. Fluoxetine and suicide: A meta-analysis of controlled trials of treatment of depression. *British Medical Journal* 303:685–92.

Beck, A. T. 1976. *Cognitive therapy and the emotional disorders*. New York: International Universities Press.

Beitman, B. D., and G. L. Klerman, (eds.). 1991. *Integrating pharmacotherapy and psychotherapy*. Washington, D.C.: American Psychiatric Press.

Benet, L. Z., J. R. Mitchell, and L. B. Sherner. 1990a. General principles. In *Goodman & Gilman's: The pharmacological basis of therapeutics*, A. G. Gilman, T. W. Rall, A. S. Nies, and P. Taylor, eds. New York: Pergamon Press.

Benet, L. Z., J. R. Mitchell, and L. B. Sherner. 1990b. Pharmacokinetics: The dynamics of drug absorption, distribution and elimination. In *Goodman & Gilman's: The pharmacological basis of therapeutics*, A. G. Gilman, T. W. Rall, A. S. Nies, and P. Taylor, eds. New York: Pergamon Press.

Bender, K. J. (ed.). 1993. Narcotic antagonist for alcoholism. *Psychotropics* 13:6–8.

Bieck, P. R., and K. Antonin. 1988. Oral tyramine pressor test and the safety of monoamine oxidase inhibitor drugs: Comparison of brofaromine and tranylcypromine in healthy subjects. *Journal of Clinical Psychopharmacology* 8:237–45.

Bleuler, M. 1968. Prognosis of schizophrenic psychoses: A summary of personal research. In *The schizophrenias*, F. Flach, ed. New York: Norton.

Bly, R. 1990. *Iron John*. Reading, Mass: Addison-Wesley Publishing.

Briggs, G. G. 1992. Drugs in pregnancy and lactation. In *Applied therapeutics: The clinical use of drugs*, 5th ed., M. A. Koda-Kimble, L. Y. Young, W. A. Kradjan, and B. J. Guglielmo, eds. Vancouver, Wash.: Applied Therapeutics.

Brotman, A. 1992. *Practical reviews in psychiatry* (audiotape). Birmingham, Ala.: Educational Reviews.

Brown, C. S., and S. G. Bryant. 1992. Major depressive disorders. In *Applied Therapeutics: The clinical use of drugs*, 5th ed, M. A. Koda-Kimble, L. Y. Young, W. A. Kradjan, and B. J. Guglielmo, eds. Vancouver, Wash.: Applied Therapeutics.

Brown, S. A., and M. A. Schuckit. 1988. Changes in depression among abstinent alcoholics. *Journal of the Study of Alcoholism* 49:412–17.

Burton, T. M. 1991. Antidepression drug of Eli Lilly loses sales after attack by sect. *Wall Street Journal*, April 19, A1–A2.

Carlson, G. A., and F. K. Goodwin. 1973. The stages of mania. *Archives of General Psychiatry* 28: 221–28.

Carpenter, W. T., T. E. Hanlon, D. W. Heinrichs, A. T. Summerfelt, B. Kirkpatrick. J. Levine, and R. W. Buchanan. 1990. Continuous versus targeted medication in schizophrenic outpatients: Outcome results. *American Journal of Psychiatry* 147:1138–48.

Cohen, L. S., V. L. Heller, and J. F. Rosenbaum. 1989. Treatment guidelines for psychotropic drug use in pregnancy. *Psychosomatics* 30:25–33.

Cornelius, J. R., P. H. Soloff, J. M. Perel, and R. F. Ulrich. 1991. A preliminary trial of fluoxetine in refractory borderline patients. *Journal of Clinical Psychopharmacology* 11:116–20.

Cowdry, R. W., and D. L. Gardner. 1988. Pharmacotherapy of borderline personality disorder. *Archives of General Psychiatry* 45:111–19.

Cowley, G., K. Springer, E. A. Leonard, K. Robins and J. Gorden, 1990. The promise of Prozac. *Newsweek* March 26:38–41.

Crutchfield, J., J. Farmer, N. H. Packard, and R. Shaw. 1986. Chaos. *Scientific American* 255:46–57.

Daro, D. 1989. *The most frequently "asked about" issues regarding child abuse and neglect*. Toledo, Ohio: NCE Foundation for the Prevention of Child Abuse.

Davidson, J., H. Kudler, R. Smith, S. L. Mahorney, S. Lipper, E. Hammett, W. B. Saunders, and J. O. Cavenar. 1990. Treatment of PTSD with amitriptyline and placebo. *Archives of General Psychiatry* 47:259–66.

Davidson, J., S. Roth, and E. Newman. 1991. Fluoxetine in post-traumatic stress disorder. *Journal of Traumatic Stress* 4:419–23.

Davis, K., R. Kahn, G. Ko, and M. Davidson. 1991. Dopamine in schizophrenia: A review and reconceptualization. *American Journal of Psychiatry*. 148:1474–84.

Deckert, G. 1985. Advances in neuro-biology. Paper presented at Continuing Education Advanced Psychiatric Update, San Francisco, Calif.

DSM-IV draft criteria, 1993. Washington D.C.: American Psychiatric Association.

Ereshefsky, L., and A. L. Richards. 1992. Psychoses. In *Applied therapeutics: The clinical use of drugs*, 5th ed., M. A. Koda-Kimble, L. Y. Young, W. A. Kradjan, B. J. Guglielmo, eds. Vancouver: Wash.: Applied Therapeutics.

Eysenck, H. J. 1965. The effects of psychotherapy: An evaluation. *Journal of Consulting Psychology* 16:319–24.

Facts and Comparisons. 1993. St. Louis, MO: Facts and Comparisons.

Fava, M., and J. F. Rosenbaum. 1991. Suicidality and fluoxetine: Is there a relationship? *Journal of Clinical Psychiatry*. 52:108–11.

Francis, A. J. 1989. *Borderline personality disorder* (audiotape). New York: Guilford Publications.

Francis, A. J., and P. H. Soloff, 1988. Treating the borderline patient with low-dose neuroleptics. *Hospital and Community Psychiatry* 39:246–48.

Frank, J. D. 1973. *Persuasion and healing*, 2nd ed. Baltimore: Johns Hopkins University Press.

Freud, S. 1895. Project for a scientific psychology, in vol. 1 of *The standard edition of the complete psychological works of Sigmund Freud*, J. Strachey, ed. London: Hogarth Press, 1953.

Freud, S. 1917. Mourning and melancholia, in vol. 14 of *The standard edition of the complete psychological works of Sigmund Freud*. London: Hogarth Press, 1957.

Gardner, D. L., and R. W. Cowdry. 1986. Positive effects of carbamazepine on behavioral dyscontrol in borderline personality disorder. *American Journal of Psychiatry* 143:519–22.

Gelenberg, A. J., and S. C. Schoonover. 1991. Bipolar disorder. In *The practitioner's guide to psychoactive drugs*, 3rd ed., A. J. Gelenberg, E. L. Bassuk, and S. C. Schoonover, eds. New York: Plenum.

Gennaro, A. R. 1980. Inorganic pharmaceutical chemistry. In *Remington's pharmaceutical sciences*, 16th ed., A. Osol, ed. Easton, Penn.: Mack.

George, A., and P. H. Soloff. 1986. Schizotypal symptoms in patients with borderline personality disorder. *American Journal of Psychiatry* 143:212–15.

Glazener, F. S. 1992. Adverse drug reactions. In *Melmon and Morrelli's clinical pharmacology: Basic principles in therapeutics* 3rd ed. D. W. Nierenberg, eds., New York: McGraw-Hill.

Goldberg, S. C., S. C. Schulz, P. M. Schulz, R. J. Resnick, R. M. Hamer, and R. O. Friedel. 1986. Borderline and schizotypal personality disorders treated with low dose thiothixene vs. placebo. *Archives of General Psychiatry* 43:680–86.

Goodman, A. 1991. Organic unit theory: The mind-body problem revisited. *American Journal of Psychiatry* 148:553–63.

Gordon, B. 1990. *I'm dancing as fast as I can*. New York: Bantam.

Hall, R., M. Popkin, R. Devaul, L. Fairlace, and S. Stickney. 1978. Physical illness presenting as psychiatric disease. *Archives of General Psychiatry* 35:1315–20.

Hansten, P. D., and J. R. Horn. 1990. Drug interaction mechanisms and clinical characteristics. In *Drug interactions and updates*. Vancouver, Wash.: Applied Therapeutics.

Hansten, P. D., and J. R. Horn. 1993. Drug interactions and updates. Vancouver, Wash.: Applied Therapeutics.

Harlow, H. F., and M. K. Harlow. 1971. Psychopathology in monkeys. In *Experimental psychopathology*, H. D. Kimmal, ed. New York: Academic Press.

Hirschfeld, R. M., and F. K. Goodwin. 1988. Mood disorders. In *The American Psychiatric Press textbook of psychiatry*, J. A. Talbott, R. E. Hales, and S. C. Yudofsky, eds. Washington D.C.: American Psychiatric Press.

Hollister, L. E. 1992. Psychiatric disorders. In *Melmon and Morrelli's clinical pharmacology: Basic principles in therapeutics*, 3rd ed., K. L. Melmon, H. F. Morrelli, B. B. Hoffman, and D. W. Nierenberg, eds. New York: McGraw-Hill.

Horowitz, M. J. 1976. *Stress response syndromes*. New York: Jason Aronson.

Jann, M. W. 1992. Anxiety. In *Applied therapeutics: The clinical use of drugs*, 5th ed., M. A. Koda-Kimble, L. Y. Young, W. A. Kradjan, and B. J. Guglielmo, eds. Vancouver, Wash.: Applied Therapeutics.

Javitt, D., and S. Zukin. 1991. Recent advances in the phencyclidine model of schizophrenia. *American Journal of Psychiatry* 148:1301–7.

Jinks, M. J., and R. H. Fuerst. 1992. Geriatric therapy. In *Applied therapeutics: The clinical use of drugs*, 5th ed., M. A. Koda-Kimble, L. Y. Young, W. A. Kradjan, and B. J. Guglielmo, eds., Vancouver, Wash.: Applied Therapeutics.

Kane, J. M. 1990. Treatment programme and long-term outcome in chronic schizophrenia. *Acta psychiatrica scandinavica* 82 (supp.) 358:151–57.

Kety, S. S. 1975. Progress toward an understanding of the biological substrates of schizophrenia. In *Genetic research in psychiatry*, R. R. Fieve, et al., eds. Baltimore: John Hopkins University Press.

Kety, S. S., D. Rosenthal, T. H. Wender, and F. Schulsinger. 1971. Mental illness in the biological and adoptive families of adopted schizophrenics. American Journal of Psychiatry 128:302–6.

Klerman, G. L., M. M. Weissman, B. J. Rounsaville, and E. Chevron. 1984. *Interpersonal psychotherapy of depression*. New York: Basic Books.

Koran, L., H. Sox, K. Marton, S. Moltzen, H. Kraemer, T. Kelsey, L. Levin, K. Imai, T. Rose, and S. Chandra. 1989. Medical evaluation of psychiatric patients: I. Results in a state mental health system. *Archives of General Psychiatry* 46:733–40.

Kraemer, G. W., M. H. Ebert, and S. R. Lake. 1984. Hypersensitivity to d-amphetamine several years after early social deprivation in rhesus monkeys. *Psychopharmacology* 82:266–71.

Kraepelin, E. 1898. *Textbook of Psychiatry*, 7th ed. (abstracted). Translated by Diefendorf. London: MacMillan 1907.

Kramer, P. D. 1993. *Listening to Prozac*. New York: Viking.

Langtry, H. D., and P. Benfield. 1990. Zolpidem: A review of its pharmacodynamic and pharmacokinetic properties and therapeutic potential. *Drug* 40:291–313.

Liebowitz, M. R., and D. F. Klein. 1979. Hysteroid-dysphoria. *Psychiatric Clinics of North America* 2:555–75.

Liebowitz, M. R., and D. F. Klein. 1981. Interrelationships of hysteroid-dysphoria and borderline personality disorder. *Psychiatric Clinics of North America*, 4:67–87.

Loebel, A. D., J. A. Lieberman, J. M. J. Alvir, D. I. Mayerhoff, S. H. Geisler, and S. R. Szymanski. 1992. Duration of psychosis and outcome in first episode schizophrenia. *American Journal of Psychiatry* 149:1183–88.

Luby, E. D., J. S. Gottlieb, B. D. Cohen, G. Rosenbaum, E. F. Domino. 1962. Model psychoses and schizophrenia. *American Journal of Psychiatry* 119:61–67

Luby, E. D., M. A. Marrazzi, and J. Kinzie 1987. Letter to the editor. *Journal of Clinical Psychopharmacology* 7:52–53

Malaspina, O., H. M. Quitkin, and C. A. Kaufmann. 1992. Epidemiology and genetics of neuropsychiatric disorders. In *The American Psychiatric Press textbook of neuropsychiatry*, S. C. Yudofsky and R. E. Hales, eds. Washington, D.C.: American Psychiatric Press.

Menninger, K. 1963. *The vital balance*. New York: Viking.

Meyer, U. A. 1992. Drugs in special patient groups: Clinical importance of genetics in drug effects. In *Melmon and Morrelli's clinical pharmacology: Basic principles in therapeutics*, 3rd ed., K. L. Melmon, H. F. Morrelli, B. B. Hoffman, and D. W. Nierenberg, eds. New York: McGraw-Hill.

Michaels, R. 1992. *Principles of psychodynamic psychotherapy*. Glendale, Calif.: *Audio Digest Psychiatry* 20 no. 13.

Nagy, L. M., C. A. Morgan, S. M. Southwick, and D. S. Charney. 1993. Open prospective trial of fluoxetine for post-traumatic stress disorder. *Journal of Clinical Psychopharmacology* 13:107–13.

Norden, M. J. 1989. Is there an effective drug treatment for borderline personality disorder? *Harvard Mental Health Letter* 6:8.

Pinsker, H., I. Kupfermann, V. Castellucci, and E. Kandel. 1970. Habituation and dishabituation of the gill-withdrawal reflex in Aplysia. *Science* 167:1740–42.

Pollock, V. E. 1992. Meta-analysis of subjective sensitivity to alcohol in sons of alcoholics. *American Journal of Psychiatry* 149:1534–38.

Post, R. M., S. R. B. Weiss, and O. Chuang. 1992. Mechanisms of action of anticonvulsants in affective disorders: Comparisons with lithium. *Journal of Clinical Psychopharmacology* 12:23S–35S.

Preston, J. D. 1993. *Depression and Anxiety Management* (audiotape). Oakland, Calif.: New Harbinger Publications.

Rabkin, J. G., F. M. Quitkin, P. McGrath, W. Harrison, and E. Tricamo. 1985. Adverse reactions to monoamine oxidase inhibitors, part II: Treatment correlates and clinical management. *Journal of Clinical Psychopharmacology* 5:2–9.

Rapoport, J. L. 1991. Recent advances in obsessive-compulsive disorder. *Neuropsychopharmacology* 5:1–10.

Rosenthal, J., A. Strauss, L. Minkoff, and A. Winston. 1986. Identifying lithium-responsive bipolar depressed patients using nuclear magnetic resonance. *American Journal of Psychiatry* 143:779–80.

Rubin, P. C. 1992. Drugs in special patient groups: Pregnancy and nursing. In *Melmon and Morrelli's clinical pharmacology: Basic principles in therapeutics*, 3rd ed., K. L. Melmon, H. F. Morrelli, B. B. Hoffman, and D. W. Nierenberg, eds. New York: McGraw-Hill.

Russell, E. W., C. Neuringer, and G. Goldstein. 1970. *Assessment of brain damage: A neuropsychological key approach*. New York: Wiley.

Sackett, G. P. 1965. Effects of rearing conditions on the behavior of the rhesus monkey. *Child Development* 36:855–68.

Safer, D. J., and J. M. Krager. 1992. Effect of a media blitz and a threatened lawsuit on stimulant treatment. *JAMA* 268:1004–7.

Schuckit, M. A., E. Gold, and C. Risch. 1987. Serum prolactin levels in sons of alcoholics and control subjects. *American Journal of Psychiatry* 144:854–59.

Schuckit, M. A., M. Irwin, and S. A. Brown. 1990. The history of anxiety symptoms among 171 primary alcoholics. *Journal of the Study of Alcoholism* 51:34–41.

Shimoda, K., T. Minowada, T. Noguchi, and S. Takahashi. 1993. Interindividual variations of desmethylation and hydroxylation of clomipramine in an Oriental psychiatric population. *Journal of Clinical Psychopharmacology* 13:181–88.

Shulman, K. I., S. E. Walker, S. MacKenzie, and S. Knowles. 1989. Dietary restriction, tyramine, and the use of monoamine oxidase inhibitors. *Journal of Clinical Psychopharmacology* 9:397–402.

Smith, D. F., and D. R. Wesson. 1983. Benzodiazepine dependency syndromes. *Journal of Psychoactive Drugs* 15:85–95.

Smith, S. S., B. F. O'Hara, A. M. Persico, D. A. Gorelick, D. B. Newlin, D. Vlahov, L. Solomon, R. Pickens, and G. R. Uhl. 1992. Genetic vulnerability to drug abuse. *Archives of General Psychiatry* 49:723–27.

Snodgrass, W. R. 1992. Drugs in special patient groups: Neonates and children. In *Melmon and Morrelli's clinical pharmacology: Basic principles in therapeutics*, 3rd ed., K. L. Melmon, H. F. Morrelli, B. B. Hoffman, and D. W. Nierenberg, eds. New York: McGraw-Hill.

Soloff, P. H., A. George, R. S. Nathan, P. M. Schulz, R. F. Ulrich, and J. M. Perel. 1986. Progress in psychopharmacology of borderline disorders. *Archives of General Psychiatry* 43:691–97.

Spiegel, R., and H. J. Aebi. 1989. *Psychopharmacology: An introduction.* Chichester, U.K.: John Wiley and Sons.

Stewart, J. W., F. J. Quitkin, and D. F. Klein. 1992. The pharmacotherapy of minor depression. *American Journal of Psychotherapy* 46:23–36.

Stone, M. H. 1988. Toward a psychobiological theory of borderline disorder. *Dissociation* 1:2-15.

Stoudemire, A., R. Frank, N. Hedemark, M. Kamlet, and D. Blazer. 1986. The economic burden of depression. *General Hospital Psychiatry* 8:387–94.

Strub, R. L., and F. W. Black. 1985. *The mental status examination in neurology,* 2nd ed. Philadelphia: F. A. Davis.

Taylor, R. L. 1990. *Distinguishing psychological from organic disorders.* New York: Springer Publishing.

Teicher, M. H., C. Glod, and J. O. Cole. 1990. Emergence of intense suicidal preoccupation during fluoxetine treatment. *American Journal of Psychiatry* 147:207–10.

Terr, L. C. 1991. Childhood traumas: An outline and overview. *American Journal of Psychiatry* 148:10–20.

Tsuang, M. T., and S. V. Faraone. 1990. *The genetics of mood disorders.* Baltimore: Johns Hopkins University Press.

Ulenhuth, E. H., H. DeWit, M. B. Balter, C. E. Johanson, and G. D. Mellinger. 1988. Risks and benefits of long term benzodiazepine use. *Journal of Clinical Psychopharmacology* 8:161–167.

van der Kolk, B. A. 1987. *Psychological trauma.* Washington, D. C.: American Psychiatric Press.

Vestal, R. E., S. C. Montamat, and C. P. Nielson. 1992. Drugs in special patient groups: The elderly. In *Melmon and Morrelli's clinical pharmacology: Basic principles in therapeutics*, 3rd ed., K. L. Melmon, H. F. Morrelli, B. B. Hoffman, and D. W. Nierenberg, eds. New York: McGraw-Hill.

Vestergaard, P., A. Amdisen, and M. Schow. 1980. Clinically significant side effects of lithium treatment. *Acta Psychiatrica Scandinavica* 62:193–200.

Ward, N. 1992. Psychopharmacology update. Pharmaceutical company presentation, Sacramento, Calif.

Watsky, E. J., and C. Salzman. 1991. Psychotropic drug interactions. *Hospital and Community Psychiatry* 42:247–56.

Weber, S. S., S. R. Saklad, and K. V. Kastenholz. 1992. Bipolar affective disorders. In *Applied therapeutics: The clinical use of drugs*, 5th ed., M. A. Koda-Kimble, L. Y. Young, W. A. Kradjan, and B. J. Guglielmo, eds. Vancouver, Wash.: Applied Therapeutics.

Weinberger, D. R., K. F. Berman, R. Suddath, and E. F. Torrey. 1992. Evidence of dysfunction of a prefrontal-limbic network in schizophrenia: A magnetic resonance imaging and regional cerebral blood flow study of discordant monozygotic twins. *American Journal of Psychiatry* 149:890–97.

Weiss, J., H. I. Glazer, and L. A. Pohorecky. 1976. Coping behavior and neurochemical changes in rats: An alternative explanation for the original "learned helplessness" experiments. In *Animal models in human psychobiology*, G. Servan and A. Kling, eds. New York: Plenum Press.

Winchel, R. M., and M. Stanley. 1991. Self-injurious behavior: A review of the behavior and biology of self-mutilation. *American Journal of Psychiatry* 148:306–317.

Winter, M. E. 1988. *Basic clinical pharmacokinetics*. Vancouver, Wash.: Applied Therapeutics.

Young, J. Z. 1987. *Philosophy and the brain*. Oxford: Oxford University Press.

Index

Note: Page numbers in italics refer to tables, lists, and figures boxed for quick reference.

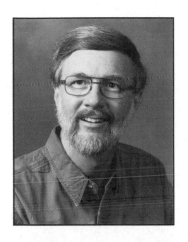

John Preston, Psy. D., is a clinical psychologist in private practice in Sacramento, California, and author of four other books, including *You Can Beat Depression* and *Growing Beyond Emotional Pain*. He has taught on the faculty of the University of California at Davis School of Medicine, and is currently the chairman of the faculty for the Professional School of Psychology in Sacramento, California.

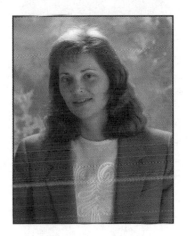

Mary C. Talaga, R.Ph., M.A. is pharmacist-in-Charge at Kaiser Psychiatric Center, Sacramento, California. She has been a pharmacist for seventeen years, specializing in psychiatric pharmacy for the last seven years. Ms. Talaga frequently gives in-service training on psycho-pharmacology and general pharmacy for school counselors and health care professionals. She is also an assistant clinical professor, Division of Clinical Pharmacy, at the University of California San Francisco School of Pharmacy.

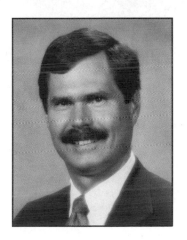

John H. O'Neal, M.D. has been a board-certified psychiatrist in private practice since 1977. A past chief of the Department of Psychiatry at Sutter Community Hospital in Sacramento, Dr. O'Neal is currently on the hospital staff. He is also an associate clinical professor of psychiatry at the University of California at Davis School of Medicine. He lectures on depression and psychopharmacology to mental health professionals, employee assistance programs, and the public. Dr. O'Neal received his M.A. in psychology from Harvard University.

Other New Harbinger Self-Help Titles